Narrative Medicine

Narrative Medicine: A Rhetorical Rx rests on the principles that storytelling is central to medical encounters between caregivers and patients and that narrative competence enhances medical competence. Thus, the book's goal is to develop the narrative competence of its reader. Grounded in the rhetorical theory of narrative that Phelan has been constructing over the course of his career, this volume utilizes a three-step method:

1 Offering a jargon-free explication of core concepts of narrative such as character, progression, perspective, time, and space.
2 Demonstrating how to use those concepts to interpret a diverse group of medical narratives, including two graphic memoirs.
3 Pointing to the relevance of those demonstrations for caregiver-patient interactions.

Narrative Medicine: A Rhetorical Rx is the ideal volume for undergraduate students interested in pursuing careers in health care, students in medical and allied health professional schools, and graduate students in the health humanities and social sciences.

James Phelan, Distinguished University Professor of English at Ohio State University, is the author, co-author, editor, or co-editor of more than 20 books, including *Narrative as Rhetoric* (1996), *Living to Tell about It* (2005), *Experiencing Fiction* (2007), *Reading the American Novel, 1920–2010* (2013), *Somebody Telling Somebody Else* (2017), and, with Matthew Clark, *Debating Rhetorical Narratology* (2020). He has been the editor of *Narrative*, the journal of the International Society for the Study of Narrative, since its inception in 1993. He has received an honorary doctorate from Aarhus University in Denmark and been elected into the Norwegian Academy of Letters and Science. In 2021 he received the Wayne C. Booth Lifetime Achievement Award from the International Society for the Study of Narrative.

Narrative Medicine
A Rhetorical Rx

James Phelan

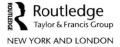
Routledge
Taylor & Francis Group

NEW YORK AND LONDON

Cover image: © Getty Images

First published 2023
by Routledge
605 Third Avenue, New York, NY 10158

and by Routledge
4 Park Square, Milton Park, Abingdon, Oxon OX14 4RN

Routledge is an imprint of the Taylor & Francis Group, an informa business

ISBN: 978-0-367-89377-4 (hbk)
ISBN: 978-0-367-89320-0 (pbk)
ISBN: 978-1-003-01886-5 (ebk)

DOI: 10.4324/9781003018865

Typeset in Bembo
by Taylor & Francis Books

For Betty Menaghan, with all my love

Contents

Figures

Acknowledgments

As anyone who has written a book knows, it is much like raising a child: it takes a village—but one that can extend across continents. I want to thank all my fellow villagers even as I give a short, incomplete list of names: Frederick Aldama, Nimisha Bajaj, Elinor Brown, Katra Byram, Matthew Clark, Angus Fletcher, Jared Gardner, Faye Halpern, Lindsay Holmgren, Stefan Iversen, Erin McConnell, Brian McHale, Brian Richardson, Amy Shuman, Richard Walsh, Robyn Warhol, and Henrik Zetterberg-Nielsen. Peter J. Rabinowitz, my long-time collaborator and conversational partner, has influenced a lot of what I say about narrative as rhetoric. Two colleagues working on Narrative Medicine have been especially important. The first is Rita Charon, the doctor/narrative theorist/Henry James scholar, whose vision and indefatigable efforts have done so much to launch and sustain the Narrative Medicine movement. Rita and her colleagues at Columbia University have made powerful interventions in both narrative studies and medical practices. Without their work, this book would not exist. Second, John Vaughn, my former colleague at Ohio State University and now the Director of Student Health Services and Assistant Vice-President of Student Affairs at Duke University. During his time in Columbus, John and I frequently co-taught an undergraduate course called Narrative and Medicine, and we co-directed a course in the College of Medicine, called Literature for Physicians: From the Page to the Bedside. John supplied the patient case history that I discuss in the first chapter. I give special thanks to Joey Ferraro, who helped greatly with the preparation of the final manuscript, including with some helpful substantive suggestions.

Finally, I dedicate this book to my wife, Betty Menaghan, whose love and support have been beyond measure for more than a half-century. What stories we can tell!

The book contains material from previous publications, much of it revised and all of it recontextualized to fit the needs and purposes of this book. I thank the publishers for permission to reprint.

Chapter 1 contains material from "Character as Rhetorical Resource: Mimetic, Thematic, and Synthetic in Fiction and Non-Fiction," *Narrative* 30 (2022): 256–263.

Chapter 5 contains material from *Somebody Telling Somebody Else: A Rhetorical Poetics of Narrative*. Columbus, OH: Ohio State University Press, 2017, pp. 206–209, 214.

Chapters 5, 8, and 11 contain material from "Toward a Rhetorical Narrative Medicine: Corpus, Close Reading, and the Cases of Oates's 'Hospice/Honeymoon' and Ward's 'On Witness and Respair.'" In *The Routledge Companion to Narrative Theory*, edited by Paul Dawson and Maria Mäkelä, 299–312. New York: Routledge, 2023.

Chapter 7 contains material from "Analepsis/Prolepsis." In *Time: Keywords*, edited by Amy Elias and Joel Burgess, 24–54. New York: NYU Press, 2016.

Chapter 9 contains material from "Irony, Ethics, and Lyric Narrative in Miriam Engelberg's *Cancer Made Me a Shallower Person*." In *Oxford Handbook to Comic Studies*, edited by Frederick Luis Aldama, 311–325. New York: Oxford University Press, 2019.

Chapter 10 contains material from "Local Fictionality within Global Nonfiction: Roz Chast's *Can't We Talk about Something More Pleasant?*" *Enthymema* 16 (2016). https://riviste.unimi.it/index.php/enthymema/article/view/7473

Preface

Narrative Medicine is a project for transforming medical practice grounded in the principle that increasing the skills of caregivers and patients as storytellers and story-listeners can improve both caregiver-patient interactions and the outcomes of medical treatment. *Narrative Medicine: A Rhetorical Rx* makes a case for the value of a rhetorical approach to the project. Given that goal, I find it appropriate here at the outset to turn a rhetorical lens on the book itself.

Conceiving of narrative as rhetoric leads to the following definition of it: somebody telling somebody else on some occasion and for some purpose(s) that something happened. Adjusting that definition because this book develops an approach rather than tells a story yields the following description: somebody modeling for a range of readers in the third decade of the twenty-first century how to improve their skills in constructing, reading, and listening to stories for the purpose of enhancing medical experiences. Let's take a closer look.

The "somebody modeling" is a narrative theorist and a (sometime) patient but not a doctor or other caregiver, and, thus, somebody who knows more about the first term in the book's title than the second. This fact means that I make many claims about narrative and how it works and almost no *specific* claims about what should happen in the clinic. I prefer to let those who face the challenges and rewards of clinical encounters—both caregivers and patients—apply the Lessons of Rhetoric as they see fit. Indeed, one of those Lessons is that tellers and audiences need to adjust their tellings and responses to the particular features of their communicative contexts. Nevertheless, I make—or, better, echo—the general claim of the Narrative Medicine movement that the encounters between patients and caregivers can be improved if both parties become better storytellers and better story-listeners. I then model the practice of rhetorical listening as I discuss a dozen remarkable stories (more on those soon). Furthermore, at the end of Chapters 3 to 10, under the subheading "Opening Out," I offer some brief, general suggestions—not prescriptions—about how caregivers and patients might take a few steps from the model analyses to their own situations.

With my references to caregivers and patients, I've already begun to gloss the phrase "range of readers." I address the book primarily to undergraduate and graduate students and their teachers in the health humanities and social sciences, to medical students and their teachers, and to doctors (including residents), nurses, and other caregivers. I realize that different segments of my large target audience are likely to want different things from the book, and that realization has influenced some of my choices in constructing it. Doctors, nurses, and other caregivers may find it difficult to find the time to work step-by-step through each chapter, but I think they can benefit by reading Chapters 1 and 2 on the rhetorical approach and then going to Chapter 11, which provides a template for Rhetorical Narrative Medicine workshops. They can then take up the other chapters as time permits. Readers who find comics an especially appealing medium may want to read Chapters 1 and 2 and then jump to Chapter 9 on graphic narrative. Readers who have special interests in particular resources of narrative—e.g., time, space, fictionality—may want to read Chapters 1 and 2 and then the chapter devoted to that resource. Other subgroups of the target audience may prefer their own alternative routes through the book.

In Chapters 1 through 10, I have sought to balance the need to be clear and accessible with the need to give enough detail about rhetorical theory to demonstrate its potential for improving our reading/listening skills. (Chapter 11 also aims to be clear and accessible but it applies rather than explicates rhetorical theory.) In Chapters 1 through 10, then, I begin with a discussion of theoretical material—about narrative as rhetoric and/or about the resources of narrative—and then show how those theoretical constructs can generate non-trivial insights into one or more narratives in my corpus. Furthermore, I typically treat each of the narratives in more than one chapter in order to demonstrate that attending to a teller's handling of multiple resources is essential to understanding their rhetorical communication—and also to suggest that I know that I am not offering the last word on any of the rich narratives I discuss.

I have chosen to work with ten short print narratives, some fictional and some nonfictional, and with two graphic memoirs. I have chosen these narratives because I believe that they collectively constitute a manageable reading list for a Narrative Medicine course, even as they come from a group of diverse authors treating a wide range of medical issues in striking ways. Here's the list in alphabetical order by author surname:

Roger Angell, "This Old Man"
Roz Chast, *Can't We Talk about Something More Pleasant?*
Edwidge Danticat, "Sunrise/Sunset"
Miriam Engelberg, *Cancer Made Me a Shallower Person*
Charlotte Perkins Gilman, "The Yellow Wallpaper"
Joyce Carol Oates, "Widow's First Year" and "Hospice/Honeymoon"
Richard Selzer, "Imelda"

Colm Toíbín, "One Minus One"
Damon Tweedy, "People Like Us" from *Black Man in a White Coat*
Jesmyn Ward, "On Witness and Respair: Personal Tragedy Followed by Pandemic"
Tobias Wolff, "Close Calls" from *In Pharaoh's Army*

I hope that these choices about my organization and my corpus will encourage teachers to use the book in a variety of ways. Teachers, you might want to put the 12 narratives on your syllabus, and then work through the book's analyses of them with your students. You might want to use those same narratives but mix and match them with the theoretical material somewhat differently: for example, where I focus on "space" in my discussion of Gilman's "The Yellow Wallpaper," you might want to give primary attention to time. Alternatively, you might want to assign the theoretical material and ask students to apply it to a different set of primary narratives. Or you might want to combine some of these strategies. Again, one Lesson of Rhetoric is that tellers and listeners should adapt their exchanges to their particular communicative contexts.

As for occasion, that is, modeling rhetorical reading for an educated audience at this point in time, I want to highlight the idea that both rhetorical narrative theory and Narrative Medicine are continually evolving enterprises. This book captures each at a moment in time, and, thus, I don't claim to be offering immutable truths about either. But I hope that what I say provides a foundation for further developments in each, including some made by users of this book.

I've already discussed the purposes of Narrative Medicine, so I'll just say a little about the phrase "skills in constructing, reading, and listening to stories." My primary focus is on reading and listening rather than constructing, but I believe that becoming adept with the former can enhance one's ability with the latter. More than that, as I explain in Chapter 2, rhetorical reading involves three steps: understanding, overstanding, and springboarding, that is, listening to reconstruct a teller's communication, stepping back from the reconstruction to assess it, and then using both the reconstruction and assessment as the basis for doing other things with the narrative. Springboarding often involves the construction of new narratives. As with any skill, the best way to improve is practice, practice, practice. For that reason and in order to suggest ways to move from understanding to overstanding and springboarding, I will end Chapters 3 through 10 with some prompts for those second and third steps of rhetorical reading. Users of this book—teachers, students, curious readers—should feel free to follow those prompts or develop their own.

1 Narrative as Rhetoric and the Art of Medicine

Why This Book

Seven reasons/beliefs/motivations:

1   Medicine is both a science and an art. As a science, and especially one whose developments are interlinked with the forward march of technology, medicine has advanced far more in the last half-century than it did in its previous history. As a result, competent twenty-first century doctors must master a large body (!) of scientific and technical knowledge. I suggest we call acquiring this information "knowing-that," as in "a cardiologist must know that some changes to the arteries are beneficial, and some are not." At the same time, however, the medical profession's focus on this knowledge and some practices that follow from it have often impeded its development as an art. To take just one example, the popularity of electronic medical records often leads to caregivers interacting more with their computers than with their patients.

2   While the science of medicine requires the acquisition of a great deal of knowing-that (about the body, about illness, about drugs and so much more), the art of medicine calls for caregivers to develop a large set of skills that I suggest we call "knowing-how." The good surgeon needs to know how to handle a scalpel. The good psychiatrist needs to know how to guide a patient to new insights about themselves and their situations. Across specialties, the art of medicine is also grounded in the art of communication based in storytelling about illness by patients to caregivers and its interpretation by those caregivers. Other communication, including shared decision-making about treatment options, has its foundation in this storytelling. From this perspective, knowing how stories work and how to read and listen to them is as foundational to the art of medicine as knowing how to use a scalpel is to the art of surgery.

3   Caregivers can acquire narrative skills by (a) learning some narrative theory, and especially some of its uses for interpreting stories, since that field of study has generated its own substantial body of knowledge about how stories work; and (b) practicing the interpretation of medical

DOI: 10.4324/9781003018865-1

narratives told outside the clinic, especially but not exclusively by sophisticated and artful storytellers. Caregivers can then apply the skills they acquire to storytelling in the clinic.

4   Caregivers who become more knowledgeable about storytelling can then use that knowledge as a ground from which to reorient their practices. The degree of such reorientation can vary from caregiver to caregiver, but one fundamental move is to shift from conceiving of patients primarily through the lenses of diagnoses and treatment plans to recognizing them as people with stories in which their illnesses exist in relation to many other events. In reorienting their practices, caregivers can forge new, more productive syntheses between medicine as a science and medicine as an art.

5   Literary narratives about medical issues provide a second, more focused sphere for the development of one's knowing-that and knowing-how. Engaging with such narratives increases one's knowledge of the complexity and diversity of human experiences of illness and treatment, and enhances one's capacity for taking on the perspectives of others and empathizing with them. Caregivers who experience such engagements are likely to become more skillful practitioners of the art of medicine.

6   Finally, when readers engage seriously with literary narratives about medical issues, that engagement may prompt additional, sometimes hard-to-classify, changes in their ways of being in the world. In other words, I believe that reading the narratives that form the corpus of examples in this book, as well as countless others that I don't discuss here, can have effects that are harder to fit neatly into the boxes of knowing-that and knowing-how but are no less consequential.

7   Patients who become knowledgeable about how narrative works can contribute to enhancing the quality of their care in various ways from becoming advocates for themselves to becoming better listeners to their caregivers and ultimately better collaborators with them.

These ideas are both shared with and influenced by other advocates of Narrative Medicine. I am deeply indebted to the work of scholars such as Arthur Frank, Kathryn Montgomery, and Rita Charon, who have done so much groundbreaking work.[1] Indeed, Charon and her colleagues at Columbia University have been such influential advocates for Narrative Medicine that it is almost impossible to overestimate their importance.[2] I see this book as contributing to the Narrative Medicine movement in two ways: (a) it sets forth a clear, coherent, and capacious conception of narrative as rhetoric that is well-suited to the goals of Narrative Medicine; and (b) it models how to deploy that conception in the practice of rhetorical reading. Because the art of communication is so central to the art of medicine, a rhetorical approach focused on tellers, audiences, occasions, and purposes provides an especially valuable route for caregivers and patients to improve their skills in the art of medicine.

I begin by reflecting on the phenomenon of narrative itself and why it is such an important mode of discourse, something that is, as Roland Barthes observes, "international, transcultural, transhistorical … simply there, like life itself" (79).

The Power of Narrative

Humans are the storytelling species. Working with a rough-and-ready definition of narrative as "an account of something that happened" (I'll offer a rhetorically oriented definition below), we can recognize that narrative is the major means by which humans make sense of our experiences in and of the world, especially our experiences of time and change. Why don't we think of time as an endless undifferentiated stream of seconds moving in a single direction and steadily accompanying our relentless sequence of experiences? Because narrative provides a way to bundle, select, and sort those seconds and those experiences into larger meaningful units that are also linked to each other. Many psychologists and philosophers contend that the story (or stories) we tell about our lives constitute our identities. I'm inclined to regard that claim as overstated (I have an identity over and above the diverse stories I tell about myself), but I also see it as supporting a more modest but still powerful one. Narrative is a mode through which we come to understand not only our experiences but also ourselves. It is, in short, a way of knowing.

Furthermore, narrative is a way of doing things in the world. Joan Didion says that "we tell ourselves stories in order to live" (11). We also tell stories in order to influence other people. The patient tells the doctor a story about their illness in order to find a way to get better. The lawyer tells a story about their client's behavior in order to persuade the jury of the client's guilt or innocence. The presidential candidate tells a story about the country's past, present, and future in order to win votes. The hopeful young woman tells a young man a story from her past in order to influence his feelings about her. The revolutionary leader tells a story about how and why things need to change in order to recruit followers. The fiction writer tells an invented story in order to interpret, evaluate, and otherwise intervene in things that have happened, are happening, or might happen in the actual world. And so on.

Because humans are the storytelling species and because narrative is a way of knowing and doing, stories are everywhere in our culture. If you're interacting with others in face-to-face conversation, or via phone calls, text messages, posts on social media, or any other way (including reading this book!), you'll inevitably be involved in telling and listening to stories. If you're following the news—local, national, or international; serious or fluffy (celebrity gossip!)—you're engaging with narratives. If you're a sports fan, you're interested in the storylines about your favorite team(s) and players (and perhaps about those you love to hate). If you're a film or television buff, you're constantly taking in and responding to narrative(s). And as I've stressed above, if you're a caregiver or a patient (or both), you're telling and listening to illness narratives. Since stories are so important and so ubiquitous, knowing how to tell and listen to them can significantly enhance our ability to navigate the world. Moreover, focusing on how to listen can yield results that we can apply to our own tellings. In short, learning how to tell and to interpret stories is an invaluable aid to our efforts to come to terms with and move forward in our world.

Knowing How, Knowing That, and Narrative as Rhetoric

Knowing how to effectively tell and listen to stories entails knowing how they work. Knowing how they work helps us recognize that a given story has some purposes rather than others. Narrative theorists since Aristotle, and especially those who have been studying stories since the 1960s, have offered countless valuable insights into their structures, techniques, and effects. Not surprisingly, however, not all theorists take the same approach. Some view narrative primarily as a textual structure that combines a what, typically called *story*, and a how, typically called *discourse*. Story includes events and existents, or, things that happen, characters, and spaces. Discourse includes perspective, voice, style, and the handling of temporality. Other theorists view narrative primarily as an ideological instrument that conveys ideas about such things as identity (including race, class, gender, ability, sexuality, nationality, and their intersections) and power relations within a culture. Still others view narrative primarily as a cognitive act, a construction and reconstruction of a mental model of a storyworld. While I find value in these (and other) approaches, I integrate their important insights within a conception of narrative as rhetoric, that is, a multi-layered purposive communication between one or more tellers and one or more audiences.[3] This approach gives rise to the following default definition: somebody telling somebody else on some occasion and for some purpose(s) that something happened. An author's choice to use fiction doubles the rhetorical situation: the author tells their audience about a narrator's telling to their audience (also called the narratee).

I label this definition a "default" because I'm aware that it does not apply to all storytellers in every telling scenario: sometimes somebody tells about something that will or might—or didn't—happen; sometimes there is no clear occasion for the telling; sometimes the teller is a collective of various agents—as in film and in drama and in graphic narratives where one artist draws the images and the other supplies the verbal narration—and so on. But specifying the default helps us recognize that the variations are typically significant. I also don't claim that this rhetorical definition is the one true characterization of narrative, the best of all possible definitions, since, again, I find that different definitions are capable of providing different useful orientations toward it.

The rhetorical definition orients us toward the relations among tellers, audiences, and purposes as a way to access narrative's capacities for both knowing and doing. This orientation in turn has consequences for how I and other rhetorical analysts go about the task of interpretation. Conceiving of narrative as rhetoric means that the goal of interpretation is more than the identification of a narrative's meanings. Instead, it is the unpacking of how the author-audience-purpose nexus generates a multi-layered communication, one that appeals to its audience's cognition, affect, and ethics as well as to the interactions among those layers. This approach to narrative communication as multi-layered makes it especially suitable for caregivers (and patients) who want to become more skillful tellers and audiences of narrative: it orients its user toward the importance of accurate perspective-taking (seeing as the author and their characters see), ethics (engaging with the values explicitly or implicitly at stake in the narrative), and affect (feelings of empathy/sympathy, desire, distaste, etc. generated by the narrative). To put this point another way, many readers turn to narrative because they want to think and feel deeply about human experiences and efforts to make sense of them. Rhetorical theory seeks to understand how narratives bring about those experiences.

Rhetorical Reading: Joyce Carol Oates's "Widow's First Year"

To illustrate these points and introduce some new ones, I turn to a case study, a short short story (aka flash fiction) by Joyce Carol Oates, published in an anthology called *Hint Fiction*. I use this study to underline the difference between ordinary listening or reading, rooted in a simple understanding of a narrative's textual surface, and rhetorical listening or reading, rooted in attention to the multiple levels of communication imbricated in the author-audience-purpose nexus.

Widow's First Year
I kept myself alive.

(73)

If we focus primarily on the seven words of this text, we are likely to conclude that it is a sparse and flat story: a simple report by the unnamed widow of one thing she did during the first year after her husband died. Furthermore, that event is implied in the title: the teller wouldn't have a "first year" if she hadn't kept herself alive. But this text-centric reading misses a lot that a focus on teller, audience, and purpose enables us to see. Indeed, this focus leads us to recognize that Oates has used her seven words to fashion a cognitively sophisticated and affectively powerful story about grief that relies on and reinforces certain ethical beliefs. First, since Oates opts for fiction, she works with two tellers and thus two tellings: she gives the title in her own voice and invents the "I" who narrates the event. Second, by juxtaposing the two tellings, Oates invites her readers to look for a synergy between them. I, for one,[4] find that synergy in a progression of readerly response: an initial act of sense making (configuration) triggered by the title, and, soon after, an act of revision (reconfiguration) triggered by the narrator's sentence. The title's designation of a "year" leads me to anticipate the recounting of multiple events—not every-thing that the widow did or experienced but certainly some of her high and low points. Thus, when I read the narrator's four-word account I'm initially disappointed, because it reports just one event and because, as noted above, that event is already implied in the title itself.

Then, however, I reflect that, if I recognize that implication, Oates must as well, and so I begin to think harder about her constructive choices. I then infer that Oates layers the widow's four-word report in several ways. First, the word "first" in the title suggests something about the *occasion* of the telling: a temporal milestone has been passed and the widow takes stock. "Widow's First 2/3/X Years" doesn't convey the same sense of significant occasion as "Widow's First Year." By highlighting the widow's agency ("I kept myself" rather than, say, "I survived"), Oates turns the apparently unremarkable report into the description of a significant achievement. The widow herself is not making a boastful claim, but Oates's framing of it suggests that the event is highly tellable and thus that the report is worthy of our attention. Second, Oates's framing leads us to recognize other possibilities: the widow might not have made it through the year; her grief was so strong that it could have killed her, either by leading her to fail to take care of herself, or, more dramatically, by leading her to commit suicide. In this way, the widow's four words mask a year-long struggle of many events, many temptations not to live, and many decisions not to succumb to those temptations. Third, the first two layers open up the affective and ethical dimensions of the story, the ways in which it engages both readers' emotions and their moral values. Through them, Oates guides me to see the widow's struggle as poignant and the positive exercise of her agency as admirable.

Having done this two-step with Oates, I can consider other consequences of the interplay between the story's two voices. The narrator is talking only about herself and is making a relatively modest claim, but Oates uses the interaction of the voices to make a stronger claim about the widow's achievement and to suggest that this widow's experience is a representative one. To be sure, Oates isn't claiming that this narrator's experience will be shared by every widow, but she is suggesting that it is not unique to this unnamed character narrator. Fur-thermore, the title highlights Oates's interest in the interaction between gender and grief and invites us to think about how likely it is that a widower, however deep his grief, would experience it or express it in these terms. In these ways, Oates thematizes the widow's experience.

All these points about Oates's strategies illuminate her purpose: she wants to offer her readers a new understanding of how powerful a widow's grief can be and how going on in the face of that grief is an impressive achievement. In these ways, "Widow's First Year" exemplifies the idea that narrative is a way of knowing and of doing.

Macro–Genre: Fiction/Nonfiction

Because Oates's story is published in an anthology called *Hint Fiction*, I have so far treated it as belonging to the genre of fiction. But let's try the thought experiment of reading it as nonfiction, and even imagine it as something Oates might have said on the occasion of her doctor asking her how she was doing a year after her husband's death. We can conduct this experiment without resorting to Oates's biography, but it gains an additional warrant when we learn that Oates became a widow in 2008 after a long, happy marriage to Raymond Smith.

I suggest that the experiment yields several interrelated results.

Result #1: The story shifts from having two voices to having just one, that of Oates herself.

Result #2: The story shifts from being Oates's act of invention designed to capture something significant about a woman's grief and coping to her act of reporting, interpreting, and evaluating her coping with her own grief on the occasion of having reached one year of widowhood. In this connection, I note that Katra Byram ("Narrative as Social Action") has recently and persuasively argued that rhetorical theory needs to give more attention to the significance of occasion for both tellers and audiences. Thus, we could think about the significance of Oates making this brief nonfictional claim three years after losing her husband. (We could also think about the significance of her choice to give voice to a fictional widow at that juncture.)

Result #3: The implications of the four-word report shift. Because Oates is talking about herself, she is careful not to brag or otherwise explicitly claim that she deserves a lot of credit for her year. In other words, the apparent understatement is ethically appropriate in this context. At the same time, she trusts that her audience will recognize what it implies about the difficulty of the year. If that audience is listening well, they will pick up on those implications and feel the affective power of Oates's statement.

Result #4: Oates's thematizing also shifts. She does not claim representative status for herself in the same way that she claims it for her invented character in the fiction, but her understatement gives her assertion a force and significance that the rhetorically attentive reader will feel.

I'll return to the relations between fiction and nonfiction later in the book, especially in the next chapter when I discuss audiences and in Chapter 10 on Fictionality, but here I want to highlight some general points about those relations within a rhetorical conception of narrative.

1   We often cannot tell the difference between fiction and nonfiction just by looking at the text itself. Instead, we often need to rely on paratextual markers such as a generic label (novel, memoir, documentary, short story, narrative essay, etc.).

2   Both fiction and nonfiction involve the author's shaping of raw material, but they differ in the author's implicit claims about the result of that

shaping. The author of fiction claims that at a global level the narrative is an invention, whereas the author of nonfiction claims that at a global level the narrative's characters and events have an extratextual existence.

3   The author of nonfiction thus makes an implicit direct truth claim about the narrative's referring to extratextual reality, whereas the author of fiction makes the implicit claim that the invention provides an indirect purchase on the actual. This difference in truth claims underlies the outrage that often follows from a revelation that a narrative purporting to be nonfiction actually includes multiple acts of invention. From this perspective, the revelation does not convert the narrative from nonfiction to fiction; instead, it converts it from truth-telling (however subjective) to lying.

The Feedback Loop: Author, Resources, Audience

Well, Oates wrote a seven-word story, and I've now written almost 1400 words about it. One conclusion to draw is that I've seriously overdone it, that the widow kept herself alive only to have me come along and murder her story by overanalyzing it!

But even if you want to draw that conclusion, I would like to point to another one that can co-exist with it—and that I believe you may find more interesting because it is more radical. I offered a short version of this conclusion above, but I now want to elaborate on and provide more support for it. Although Oates's seven-word text, like the texts of most other written narratives, appears to be what determines our interpretations—after all the text is what's most prominently in front of us—that text itself is just one element of a feedback loop that also involves authorial agency and readerly response and that is itself governed by authorial purposes. In other words, understanding Oates's story involves attending to all three elements, and attending to one can shed light on the functions of the others—and attending to the whole loop can be a way to test our initial hypotheses about those functions. For example, when I checked my initial feeling of disappointment (readerly response) against my sense of why Oates would use only her four-word report (authorial agency in relation to textual phenomena and possible purposes), I revised my understanding and thus my response. At the same time, when I considered the difference between "I kept myself alive" and "I survived" (textual phenomena), I felt more confident that I understood Oates's purposes, and that understanding further influenced my readerly response.

Going further in this direction, I suggest that viewing narrative as rhetoric leads to a model of narrative communication that identifies author(s) and audience(s) as two constants and then a wide array of resources through which the constants connect with each other. These resources include all the traditional elements of narrative (e.g., event, character, time, space, perspective, and so on) as well as other resources that are not always given prominence (e.g., juxtapositions, segmentivity, occasions for telling). In *Somebody Telling Somebody Else* (2017) I sketched the Author—Resources—Audience

(ARA) model this way (though here I've added some resources to the middle column):

Chart of Constants and Variables in Narrative Communication

Author	↔	Resources	↔	Audience
Actual/Implied[5]		Occasion		Authorial and Actual
		Paratexts		
		Fictionality/Nonfictionality		
		Genre		
		Narrator(s)		
		Event		
		Plot		
		Progression		
		Characters		
		Perspective		
		Voice		
		Style		
		Segmentivity		
		Space		
		Temporality		
		Arrangement/Gaps		
		Narratee/Narrative Audience		
		Intertextual References		
		Ambiguities		
		Etc.		

(26)

In any given narrative, authors will rely on some resources more than others, and even those resources that are almost always deployed will be used in some ways rather than others. Thus, for example, Oates foregrounds narrator, voice, and temporality, and does not deploy space. The "Etc." in the middle column of the chart is designed to signify not only that the list of resources can be expanded but also that constructing a fixed comprehensive list is less important than understanding the feedback loop among authorial agency, textual phenomena, and readerly response.

As the book proceeds, I will dive more deeply into authors, audiences, and especially the resources of that middle column and the roles they can play in the feedback loops of narrative communication. But here at our beginning, I want to emphasize that all the terms and concepts I have presented in this chapter—this chart, the definition of narrative, the notions of configuration and reconfiguration, the account of the relations between fiction and nonfiction, and so on—are not ends in themselves but rather a means to give us greater understanding of and access to narrative as a way of knowing and doing that has the capacity to make us think and feel deeply.

Narrative Medicine: Literary Narratives, Rhetorical Reading, and Patients' Stories

Having read this far, you may very well have some questions about the relevance of all this literary analysis to caregiver-patient interactions. There is, after all, only one Joyce Carol Oates, and we can assume that even she would give her caregivers more than seven words to work with. So far, I have been emphasizing the idea that using a rhetorical conception of narrative can make one a better teller/listener of narrative and that working with literary narratives can sharpen those skills. Those ideas will remain central to the work of this book. At the same time, I want to show at the outset how a rhetorical approach to non-literary narratives by patients can offer caregivers a powerful framework for analyzing them.

As I noted above, almost every clinical interaction rests upon the foundation of somebody telling somebody else on some occasion and for some purpose(s) that something happened. Medicine has recognized this foundation in its formalized approach to clinical storytelling, but I suggest that conceiving of narrative as rhetoric can productively build on this foundation. Before seeing their first patient, health care providers are typically taught a very specific way to capture patients' stories and convey them to others. This formalized narrative structure plays a large role in determining how a caregiver elicits and interprets patients' stories, and it has evolved to meet the primary goal of conveying necessary clinical information as efficiently as possible, as the following outline indicates.

Chief Complaint (CC): The reason for the patient's visit to the health care provider, *in the patient's own words*.

History of Present Illness (HOPI): A description of the patient's present illness in chronological order from the time the patient first became aware of the illness (or changes from the previous clinical encounter) to the present. The HOPI should include the following elements:

- Location
- Quality (aching, burning, sharp, stabbing, dull)
- Severity
- Duration
- Timing (gradual or sudden onset; episodic or constant)
- Context (situations or activities in which symptoms occur or resolve)
- Modifying factors (things that make symptoms better or worse)
- Associated signs and symptoms

Review of Symptoms (ROS): A list of questions arranged by body systems to elicit further information/symptoms not included in the HOPI.

- Constitutional
- Ear/nose/throat
- Eyes
- Cardiovascular
- Respiratory
- Gastrointestinal
- Genitourinary
- Musculoskeletal
- Skin
- Neurological
- Psychiatric
- Hematological/lymph
- Endocrine

Past Medical History: The patient's current medical diagnoses, medications, past surgeries.

Family History: Significant medical conditions in the patient's family members.

Social History: Marital status, occupation, gender identity, substance use (alcohol, tobacco, illicit drugs), sexual history.

Physical Examination:

Laboratory or Imaging Data:

Assessment: The clinician's synthesis of all of the above narrative information and supporting data culminating in a *differential diagnosis*, a list of possible causes for the patient's current condition.

Plan: A description of next steps needed for the diagnosis (additional testing, referrals to consulting clinicians) and treatment (medications, therapies, counseling, education) of the patient.

Now let's take the story of a hypothetical patient and show how a caregiver would go from that story to filling out the standard structure and then compare the results with a rhetorical reading of that story.

> Doc, I've been having chest pains every so often for about the last year. At first it was happening only occasionally, maybe once every month to six weeks, but in the last five weeks or so, I've been having these pains more frequently. They last for maybe 10 to 15 minutes, and they hurt like hell, right in the area of my heart. I haven't been able to identify what triggers them, though sometimes they come on when I'm working out. Sometimes they also make me sick to my stomach and a little dizzy. My wife tries to stay calm during these episodes, but I can tell that they just freak her out. Her response makes me hate them even

more, but then I think that such a reaction can't be good for my heart. I've been under some stress at work, but that's been true since I started my job about four years ago, and I've never had an episode at work. I'm worried that something serious is going on with my heart.

CC (Chief Complaint): "Chest pain."

HOPI (History of Present Illness): James Rowland is a 44-year-old male who presents today for evaluation of chest pain. This is a recurrent problem, occurring approximately once a month for the past year. Recently increasing in frequency. Episodes come on suddenly and last approximately 10 minutes. The pain is described as sharp, left-sided, without radiation into the left arm or neck. These episodes seem to occur during physical exertion, are aggravated by caffeine intake, and have been gradually worsening. Associated symptoms include heart racing, dizziness, malaise/fatigue, and nausea. Patient denies chest pressure, coughing, diaphoresis, fever, irregular heartbeat, shortness of breath, syncope, vomiting, weakness, or anxiety.

ROS (Review of Symptoms):

Constitutional: Positive for malaise/fatigue. Negative for diaphoresis and fever.

Respiratory: Negative for cough and shortness of breath.

Cardiovascular: Positive for palpitations. Negative for chest pain and syncope.

Gastrointestinal: Positive for nausea. Negative for vomiting.

Neurological: Positive for dizziness. Negative for weakness.

Psychiatric/behavioral: The patient is not nervous/anxious.

Past Medical History:

Diagnoses: Hypertension, type II diabetes, obstructive sleep apnea.

Previous surgeries: Inguinal hernia repair, right ACL repair.

Medications: Metformin 1000mg PO BID; Losartan 50mg PO QD; Vitamin B-12 1000mcg PO QD; Atorvastatin 40mg PO QD; Tresiba 26u SQ QD.

Allergies: NKDA (no known drug allergies).

Family History: Mother with diabetes, breast CA [cancer]; father with hypertension and MI [myocardial infarction] in his 50s.

Social History: Patient is married and monogamous; works as a claims analyst in an insurance office. Denies the use of cigarettes or smokeless tobacco. Drinks about 4 cups of coffee per day. Consumes approximately 4.0 standard drinks of alcohol per week. Denies the use of illicit drugs. Does not regularly exercise.

Physical Examination:

Vitals:

- BP: 146/73
- Pulse: 93
- Resp: 20
- Temp: 37.2 °C (99 °F)
- Weight: 120.5kg (265 lb.)
- Height: 178 cm (5' 10")
- Pain Scale: 0—No pain
- Body mass index is 38.00 kg/m².

Constitutional: Well-nourished, obese body habitus in no apparent distress.

Neck: Normal range of motion; supple; no thyromegaly present.

Cardiovascular: Regular rate and rhythm; normal S1, S2; no murmurs, rubs, gallops.

Pulmonary/chest: Effort normal and breath sounds normal. No respiratory distress. No wheezes, rales, or rhonchi. No chest wall tenderness.

Musculoskeletal: Normal range of motion, no tenderness or edema.

Lymphadenopathy: No cervical L/A.

Skin: No rash noted.

Psychiatric: Normal mood and affect; normal behavior; normal thought content.

Lab/Imaging Data:

Urinalysis: Within normal limits, no ketones.

ECG 12-lead: No evidence of acute ischemic or dysrhythmic pathology.

Chest X-ray: No acute cardiopulmonary abnormalities noted.

Assessment: 44-year-old male with typical chest pain without syncope. Differential diagnosis includes ischemic heart disease (stable angina); medication side effect; caffeine side effect; acute anxiety episodes; cardiac dysrhythmia.

Plan: No evidence of acute ischemic or dysrhythmic cardiac pathology necessitating emergency evaluation at today's visit. Given patient's risk factors (atypical symptoms of angina; diabetes; sedentary lifestyle; significant family history), recurrent nature of symptoms and their association with exertion, will refer to cardiology for urgent evaluation. Patient advised to decrease caffeine intake (taper down gradually to avoid rebound headache) and maintain good hydration status. Patient advised to seek immediate medical evaluation if symptoms return, or he develops chest pain or shortness of breath.

This plan was discussed with the patient and all questions were answered. There were no further concerns. Follow up as indicated, or sooner should any new problems arise, if conditions worsen, or if he is otherwise concerned.

Return if symptoms worsen or fail to improve.

A Rhetorical Reading of Rowland's Narrative

I start by emphasizing that a rhetorical narrative approach is meant not to replace traditional clinical documentation but rather to add value to it. Clinical write-ups have evolved to efficiently convey large amounts of important clinical information in an increasingly specialized and complex health care system, and they're grounded in the principle that such efficient information-gathering is the best means to the ends of accurate differential diagnosis and effective treatment. A rhetorical approach shares those ends, but it adds one more, and, in so doing, it also proposes to shift the means. The additional purpose is to have the clinical encounter be one in which the caregiver and patient develop a relationship that goes beyond the efficient exchange of information. Even as the relationship remains professional and guided by the other purposes of diagnosis and treatment, it is also one in which each can and should recognize the individuality and distinctiveness of the other. Furthermore, that recognition can have consequences for diagnosis and treatment.

From the perspective of a rhetorical approach, the standard focus on information has the effect of downplaying the patient's story, of reducing the complexity of their experience to the list of symptoms and to quantifiable measures of various kinds (vitals, lab results, and so on). By giving more attention to Rowland's story, the particulars of his experience, and to the elements of narrative he uses in telling it, the rhetorical approach re-situates that valuable information within a broader context that makes possible better patient outcomes. Such outcomes may stem from a different, more accurate diagnosis and/or from a less instrumental relationship between caregiver and patient that influences the patient's engagement with the treatment plan.

Let me substantiate these points by showing how a rhetorical approach can add value to the caregiver's account of Rowland's story. Following the ARA model, I pay particular attention to author(s) and audience(s), and, from the list of resources, to voice, character, and time.

Author

Obviously, Rowland is the author of his story and the caregiver the author of the clinical narrative. But since the caregiver relies on Rowland's telling as the basis for theirs, we can look for signs of Rowland's voice in their account, beyond the Chief Complaint ("chest pains"), which is scripted into the structure. Strikingly, that phrase is the only one taken verbatim from

Rowland's story. Instead, his descriptions get translated into standard intake language, e.g., "they hurt like hell" becomes "The pain is described as sharp, left-sided, without radiation into the left arm or neck." In this way, the agency of the storytelling passes from Rowland to the caregiver. (Some of the details in the clinical narrative must come from Rowland's answers to the caregiver's follow-up questions, but, for my purposes, I don't find it necessary to do a deep dive into those details.)

Even though every symptom conveyed in the narrative belongs to Rowland, the clinician is the one writing about those symptoms and therefore shaping them into their interpretation of his condition. In that sense, the question, "whose story is it?" hangs over the whole clinical narrative. Presumably, everyone would want to answer this crucial question by saying "Rowland's." But a rhetorical analysis indicates that the standard form of the clinical narrative actually moves ownership from Rowland to the caregiver. One simple adjustment would be to have the History of Present Illness and other relevant sections of the narrative include more representation of the patient's actual voice.[6] Beyond that adjustment, thinking rhetorically about the situation emphasizes that Rowland is the ultimate owner of the story, since it's his telling that forms the basis of everything else. Ensuring that the patient retains ownership of the story provides a sound foundation for ethical decisions about treatment and, thus, for optimal care.

A rhetorical analysis of audiences, to which I now turn, indicates why it's so easy for the patient to lose ownership of their story.

Audiences

I will say more about the rhetorical model of audiences in the next chapter, so here I focus on that part of the model most relevant to Rowland's story. There are two main audiences in nonfiction—the actual and authorial. The **actual audience** is any real person who reads/listens to/views a narrative and brings their own ideas and values to that experience. The **authorial audience** is the one that the author projects. That projection typically combines what authors know about some actual readers and what they want their hypothetical readers to know and do in order to understand their communications.

In Rowland's story, then, the caregiver is the actual audience, even as Rowland shapes it according to his assumptions about the best way to get across to them just what's been happening. Thus, for example, we can see him going from the colloquial "hurts like hell" when he describes his pain to the more formal language of "identify what triggers" it, when he takes up the issue of causation. If he had a different idea of his target audience, he'd likely use different phrasing for both parts of the story.

In the caregiver's account, the actual audience is anyone who reads it—another clinician, the patient himself, a family member, an insurance claims processor, a health science student on a rotation, you, or anyone else reading this book.

But who is the authorial audience? This is a more complex question, because clinical narratives serve multiple distinct purposes, and therefore clinicians write them with multiple authorial audiences in mind. The primary authorial audience is other clinicians, and that feature of the rhetorical situation goes a long way toward determining the emphasis on information in the clinical narrative about Rowland. His caregiver writes with the purpose of conveying to other potential caregivers the details about his complaint they most need to know, whether they will be the cardiologist whom Rowland visits next, the doctor in the Emergency Room where Rowland might be taken when his chest pains become more acute, a partner in the same practice who sees Rowland in the writer's absence, or someone else.

But clinical narratives have other target audiences and serve other important purposes. They are legal documents, and the primary source of information for potential litigation that may arise from adverse patient outcomes. Therefore, clinicians are also writing for potential lawyers and judges who may read their narratives. In fact, it is ingrained in physicians early on in their training that "if it isn't documented, it didn't happen," and to "write your clinical notes as if you will be reading them out loud in a courtroom." The clinician writing about Rowland has learned these lessons well.

In the United States, clinical narratives are also the primary determination of, if, and how much a health care provider will be reimbursed for their services. In this sense, the medical narrative's function is to serve as a bill of sale. Indeed, given the importance of health insurance in the US medical system, one can plausibly argue that the most consequential authorial audience for current clinicians is their hypothetical claims processors for health insurance companies. Clinicians must write their narratives so that this projected audience will respond by saying, "yes, we cover that." The clinical narrative about Rowland would produce such a response in most claims processors.

Finally, patients themselves have become an increasingly important authorial audience for the writers of clinical narratives. Until recently, patients did not have access to their own medical records. Due to the work of patient advocacy groups, and technological advancements in electronic health records that make sharing documentation easier, patients are now often able to read clinical narratives about themself. While Rowland might pause over some of the caregiver's translations of his language, he would presumably recognize it as his.

The clinical narrative about Rowland suggests that it is possible, though not easy, to write a document that effectively addresses these multiple audiences. But a rhetorical analysis also indicates that, with so many authorial audiences to address, the caregiver almost naturally transfers ownership of the story from the patient to themselves. After all, the caregiver, not the patient, is the one who will be held responsible for any problems by the other clinicians, the lawyers and judges, the claims processors, and even the patient. How, then, can the clinician square the need to address all these audiences with the ethical principle of ensuring that the patient still owns the story of their illness? A rhetorical analysis suggests that the clinician should recognize the need for *two stories*—their own and the patient's—and that each has a distinct purpose and function. The caregiver's story is the one serving diverse purposes for its diverse authorial and actual audiences. The patient's story is the one that should be given pride of place in the caregiver-patient relationship.

Let's consider some of the other differences between the clinician's and Rowland's narrative by focusing on how each uses the resources of character and time.

Character and Time

In the clinician's story Rowland is simultaneously a particular person—in rhetorical terms, he is a character with a strong mimetic component—and part of a larger group, that is, he has a thematic component. The caregiver's narrative ultimately gives more weight to that thematic component. Indeed, the thrust of that narrative is to replace the initial mimetic understanding of Rowland as an individual patient with a thematic understanding of him as a member of the larger set of patients at risk for serious heart disease. Thus, the clinician focuses on symptoms and possible proximate causes (exertion, caffeine, etc.). Understanding the clinician's handling of character this way sheds additional light on why they translate "hurts like hell" into pain that is "sharp, left-sided, without radiation into the left arm or neck."

Rowland's story does not make such thematizing moves but, given its occasion and purpose, a rhetorical analysis of it would. Differential diagnosis is one way of thematizing an individual patient. Nevertheless, consistent with the principle that Rowland owns the story of his illness, the rhetorical analyst would not want to *replace* the mimetic with the thematic, but instead retain an awareness of Rowland's individuality and the particular details of his situation. In so doing, a rhetorical analyst would consider elements of his story that fall out of the clinician's account, especially elements that are only tangential to the report of symptoms. The most salient of these are occasion and time. The rhetorical analyst would home in on what it means for Rowland to be telling this story this way on this visit, and ask how it relates to previous storytelling on previous visits. With time, the rhetorical analyst would attend to Rowland's downplaying of his stress at work and think about it in a way that Rowland does not. Where Rowland fails to see a connection to his chest pains, the rhetorically oriented caregiver would note the duration of the stress—its persistence over time—and consider the hypothesis that it is a contributing factor to his chest pains. As a result, the treatment plan would involve some discussion about possible ways to reduce that stress.

Over and above these details of diagnosis, the caregiver who consistently sends the signal that Rowland himself matters as much as the differential diagnosis is far more likely to have Rowland follow the treatment plan than the caregiver whose primary focus is that diagnosis. In this way, reading Rowland's story rhetorically can have real consequences for his treatment.

Plan for the Book

The rest of this book is designed to expand its readers' knowledge about narrative as rhetoric (knowing-that) and to enhance its readers' skills of listening to and analyzing narrative in general and medical narratives in particular (knowing-how). Towards those ends, I have chosen to work with a set of diverse narratives, fictional and nonfictional, that address a wide range of medical issues and that raise a wide range of questions about how their authors individually and collectively use the resources of narrative to accomplish their purposes. As noted in the Preface, here's the list in alphabetical order by author surname:

Roger Angell, "This Old Man"
Roz Chast, *Can't We Talk about Something More Pleasant?*
Edwidge Danticat, "Sunrise/Sunset"
Miriam Engelberg, *Cancer Made Me a Shallower Person*
Charlotte Perkins Gilman, "The Yellow Wallpaper"
Joyce Carol Oates, "Widow's First Year" and "Hospice/Honeymoon"
Richard Selzer, "Imelda"
Colm Tóibín, "One Minus One"
Damon Tweedy, "People Like Us" (Chapter 1 from *Black Man in a White Coat*)
Jesmyn Ward, "On Witness and Respair: Personal Tragedy Followed by Pandemic"
Tobias Wolff, "Close Calls" (Chapter 4 from *In Pharaoh's Army*)

The next chapter goes further into the rhetorical conception of narrative by discussing some additional principles of rhetorical reading and describing its three steps: understanding (reading as a member of the author's target audience), overstanding (assessing that reading), and springboarding (making connections between the understanding and overstanding of the narrative with other things that matter to an actual reader). In Chapters 3 through 10, I will focus on the activity of understanding and will proceed by pairing rhetorical theory's conception of one or more key resources of narrative with one or more of the narratives in the corpus. The rhetorically inflected account of the resources provides a framework for exploring how the authors use them, even as those uses further illuminate the nature and possible functions of the resources. At the end of each chapter, I will offer some brief reflections on the relevance of the work of understanding for medical encounters (in segments I call "Opening Out") and some prompts for overstanding and springboarding.

More specifically, Chapters 3 and 4 take up narrative progression and character, with Chapter 3 focused on Selzer's "Imelda," a narrative marked by a change in the protagonist's character, and Chapter 4 focused on Tóibín's "One Minus One," a portrait narrative in which the progression is organized around the revelation of a character in a fixed situation. Chapter 5 addresses Tellers (authors, narrators, and characters) in connection with Tweedy's "People Like Us" and Oates's "Hospice/Honeymoon." It also offers a brief analysis of a passage from Joan Didion's *The Year of Magical Thinking* (the only appearance of Didion's memoir in this book, which is why I don't list it as part of my main corpus). Chapter 6 discusses voice and perspective briefly in Gilman's "Yellow Wallpaper" and Angell's "This Old Man" and more extensively in Danticat's "Sunrise/Sunset." Chapter 7 turns to time in connection with Wolff's "Close Calls" and Angell's "My Old Man." Chapter 8 explores space in connection with Oates's "Hospice/Honeymoon" and Gilman's "Yellow Wallpaper." Chapter 9 moves from print to graphic narrative with Chast's *Can't We Talk?* and Engelberg's *Cancer Made Me Shallower* as case studies. Chapter 10 takes up cross-border traffic between fictionality and nonfictionality in Wolff and Chast. I conclude the book in Chapter 11 by presenting a template for Rhetorical Narrative Medicine workshops using Ward's "On Witness and Respair" as the focal text.

Our next step, then, is to explore what it means to be a rhetorical reader/listener.

Notes

1 See the books by these scholars listed in the Works Cited.
2 In addition to her scholarship, Charon has been the prime mover behind the creation and flourishing of the MA program in Narrative Medicine at Columbia. She eminently deserved the honor of being invited to deliver the 2018 Jefferson Lecture in the Humanities at the Kennedy Center in Washington, DC, which she titled "To See the Suffering: The Humanities Have What Medicine Needs." https://edsitem ent.neh.gov/media-resources/2018-jefferson-lecture-dr-rita-charon.
3 In this book, I typically use the term "rhetorical theory" and "narrative as rhetoric" rather than "rhetorical narratology" because I want to indicate the affinity of the approach with rhetorical thinking more generally, and because I know that some people have negative associations with "narratology." But I will not object if some readers find "rhetorical narratology" an appropriate term for the approach I take here.
4 Since I don't claim that all readers, even all rhetorical readers, process narratives in exactly the same way, I will use the first-person here to describe my sense of the author-audience-purpose nexus. At the same time, I would hope that other readers can recognize that my account does offer a plausible hypothesis about that nexus. I'll return to this issue of shared experiences and interpretations in the next chapter.
5 Narratologists have debated whether to use the terms "actual author" and "implied author" to distinguish between the biographical person in general and the version of themselves that the writer constructs in the text. If we so

distinguish, then we would say that the same writer can construct different implied authors in different works (for example, John Donne constructs a different version of himself in his seduction poem "The Flea" than he does in his holy sonnets). For our purposes, however, this debate is beside the main point: the somebody who tells is the agent who constructs the text and I shall refer to them as "author."

6 Sometimes of course a patient will be unable to tell their own story. Such situations require important adjustments about how doctor and patient communicate (through a third party, via hand signals, or something else), but they typically make the caregiver's listening even more crucial.

Works Cited

Barthes, Roland. "Introduction to the Structural Analysis of Narratives." In *Image, Music, Text*, edited and translated by Stephen Heath, 79–125. New York: Hill and Wang, 1977.

Byram, Katra. "Narrative as Social Action: Making Rhetorical Narrative Theory Accountable to Context." *Poetics Today* 43, 3 (2022), 455–78.

Charon, Rita. *Narrative Medicine: Honoring the Stories of Illness*. New York: Oxford University Press, 2007.

Charon, Rita. "To See the Suffering: The Humanities Have What Medicine Needs." Jefferson Lecture in the Humanities. https://edsitement.neh.gov/media-resources/2018-jefferson-lecture-dr-rita-charon (Accessed 15 February 2022).

Charon, Rita, Sayantani DasGupta, Nellie Hermann, Craig Irvine, Eric R. Marcus, Edgar Rivera Colon, Danielle Spencer, and Maura Spiegel. *The Principles and Practice of Narrative Medicine*. New York: Oxford University Press, 2016.

Didion, Joan. *The White Album*. New York: Farrar, Straus, and Giroux, 1979.

Frank, Arthur. *Letting Stories Breathe: A Socio-Narratology*. Chicago, IL: University of Chicago Press, 2010.

Frank, Arthur. *The Wounded Storyteller*, 2nd ed. Chicago, IL: University of Chicago Press, 2013 [1995].

Montgomery, Kathryn. *Doctors' Stories: The Narrative Structure of Medical Knowledge*. Princeton: Princeton University Press, 1993.

Montgomery, Kathryn. *How Doctors Think: Clinical Judgment and the Practice of Medicine*. New York: Oxford University Press, 2005.

Oates, Joyce Carol. "Widow's First Year." In *Hint Fiction*, edited by Robert Swartwood, 73. New York: W.W. Norton & Company, 2011.

Phelan, James. *Somebody Telling Somebody Else: A Rhetorical Poetics of Narrative*. Columbus, OH: The Ohio State University Press, 2017.

2 Principles and Activities of Rhetorical Reading

Understanding, Overstanding, and Springboarding

Rhetorical Reading and the Experience of Narrative

In this chapter, I revisit and dig deeper into a set of claims I made in Chapter 1: "many readers turn to narrative because they want to think and feel deeply about human experiences." Rhetorical theory sees ethical engagement as central to such thoughts and feelings. More than that, its project is to unpack how and why narrative evokes such thoughts and feelings. These claims point to some underlying principles of rhetorical reading even as they lead to additional questions that I find important to address before I go further. Here are the principles:

1   Rhetorical reading prioritizes the experience of reading narrative, the ways that experience evokes emotion and thought as well as engagement with ethical issues. Consequently, it seeks to reason back from experience to its causes in the teller's construction of the narrative.

2   Methodologically, then, rhetorical reading works in an a posteriori rather than an a priori fashion. That is, rhetorical critics do not begin their analyses with entrenched ideas about what narratives should do or how narrative construction should work, but rather remain open to the variety of ways, old and new, that tellers construct their narratives. Among other things, the commitment to an a posteriori method means that rhetorical readers respond to most claims that "narrative always is or does X" by saying "narrative sometimes is or does X and sometimes it isn't or doesn't."

3   Rhetorical reading's interest in occasion means that it is interested in the historical contexts of telling and the ways they influence both the production and reception of narratives. As we saw with "Widow's First Year" in Chapter 1, the influence of occasion can be manifested in both a narrator's telling and an author's telling.

4   As noted in Chapter 1, rhetorical reading's focus on feeling and thinking means that it orients itself to the multiple levels of narrative communication, especially to affect, ethics, and thematics.

DOI: 10.4324/9781003018865-2

5   The focus on feeling, thinking, and ethical engagement influences rhetorical theory's model of audiences and its approach to kinds of readerly interest. I will elaborate on these influences below.

6   Rhetorical theory identifies three distinct steps of rhetorical reading: understanding, overstanding, and springboarding. The first four principles help unpack the fundamental activity of understanding, and because it is fundamental it will be the main focus of this book. Overstanding is the second step of rhetorical reading, and it involves assessing one's understanding—positively, negatively, or some combination of the two—and the reasons for and consequences of that assessment. Springboarding is the third step, and it involves using the narrative as a launching point for explorations—ideas, feelings, judgments, possible connections to text-adjacent issues—by individual readers that they likely would not have made, or would have made differently, without the steps of understanding and overstanding. Narrative Medicine Workshops based in rhetorical theory take their participants through these three steps.

I will say more about overstanding and springboarding later in this chapter, and at the end of each subsequent chapter I will offer some prompts for each of these activities. Finally, in Chapter 11, I will lay out a template for Rhetorical Narrative Medicine workshops, using Jesmyn Ward's "On Witness and Respair" as the main text.

Here are the questions that these principles often raise for those who are new to rhetorical theory, all of them about understanding:

1   Whose experiences does rhetorical reading prioritize?
2   In giving so much weight to reading in the authorial audience, does rhetorical reading risk claiming too much certainty about authors' intentions? Does it seek to impose a standard of "one right reading" that is both epistemologically and ethically untenable?
3   Aren't there other valuable things to do in response to narratives than read them rhetorically?

I'll take up these questions in order.

Question 1. Whose experiences does rhetorical reading prioritize?

The short answer is the subset of actual readers who seek to join the authorial audience, that is, the author's target audience. More formally, the authorial audience is the set of the author's ideal addressees, readers who are able to fully understand the author's rhetorical communication as the author wishes. As noted in Chapter 1, authorial audiences are typically a hybrid of what authors know about some actual readers and what they want their hypothetical readers to know and do in order to understand their communications. This conception of the authorial audience points to the importance of the occasion for the telling: what would this teller in this context expect and want the target audience to know? Saying that rhetorical reading is interested in the experiences of actual readers who want to be members of the author's target audience acknowledges upfront that not all readers want to practice rhetorical reading. I think that's a good thing. Different kinds of reading, rooted in different concepts of narrative, can offer different kinds of valuable knowledge about both narrative in general and individual narratives in particular. As also noted in Chapter 1, rhetorical reading's claim is not that it is the only, the best, or even the most comprehensive approach to narrative analysis, but rather that it is well-suited to account for the experience of reading and that its focus on the author-audience-purpose nexus fits well with the project of Narrative Medicine.

The longer answer is one that takes us further into rhetorical theory's model of audiences. This model in turn prompts some further consideration of the differences between fiction and nonfiction. Consider the following two passages, the first from Charlotte Perkins Gilman's short story "The Yellow Wallpaper," the second from Roger Angell's nonfictional narrative essay, "This Old Man."

> I wish I could get well faster.
> But I must not think about that. This paper looks to me as if it *knew* what a vicious influence it had!
> There is a recurrent spot where the pattern lolls like a broken neck and two bulbous eyes stare at you upside-down.
> I get positively angry with the impertinence of it and the ever-lastingness. Up and down and sideways they crawl, and those absurd, unblinking eyes are everywhere. There is one place where two breadths didn't match, and the eyes go all up and down the line, one a little higher than the other.
>
> (132)

> Like many men and women my age, I get around with a couple of arterial stents that keep my heart chunking. I also sport a minute plastic seashell that clamps shut a congenital hole in my heart, discovered in my early eighties. The surgeon at Mass General who fixed up this PFO (a patent foramen ovale—I love to say it) was a Mexican-born character actor in beads and clogs, and a fervent admirer of Derek Jeter. Counting this procedure and the stents, plus a passing balloon angioplasty and two or three false alarms, I've become sort of a table potato, unalarmed by the X-ray cameras swooping eerily about just above my naked body in a darkened and icy operating room; there's also a little TV screen up there that presents my heart as a pendant ragbag attached to tacky ribbons of veins and arteries. But never mind. Nowadays, I pop a pink beta-blocker and a white statin at breakfast, along with several lesser pills, and head off to my human-wreckage gym, and it's been a couple of years since the last showing.

In these passages, rhetorical readers find two first-person narrators who are concerned about the state of their health. Rhetorical readers also find that the passages offer two significantly different reading experiences. The first source of those differences is that Gilman's story is fiction and Angell's piece is nonfiction. These macro-generic frames mean that rhetorical readers understand character and situation in "The Yellow Wallpaper" as invented, and character and situation in "This Old Man" as referring to extratextual realities. With "Wallpaper," rhetorical readers automatically assume that the invention functions as *an indirect way* to intervene in the real world. As they attend to the occasion of the telling, rhetorical readers recognize that Gilman uses the invention of her character narrator to expose the horrors of the rest cure commonly prescribed for women in nineteenth-century America and to link that exposure with a critique of the patriarchal ideology that underlies the cure. Her rhetorical readers come away with a new understanding of how the patriarchy operated then and how its oppression so often had a benign face. With "This Old Man," rhetorical readers automatically assume that its referentiality functions as a direct way to intervene in the world. As they read and pay attention to the occasion of his telling— a 2014 piece in *The New Yorker*—they recognize that Angell wants to testify to and capture key aspects of what it's like to be alive in one's 90s at this point in history.

Rhetorical theory's model of audiences seeks to account for the different reading experiences offered by the two narratives. With "The Yellow Wallpaper," rhetorical readers seek to enter not just the authorial audience but also the narrative audience. With "This Old Man," rhetorical readers seek to enter only one, the authorial. Here's why.

The explanation starts with the experience of double consciousness that accompanies reading fiction. Readers develop emotions about fictional characters and their experiences and readers sometimes take on beliefs that apply only to the fictional world (e.g., magic exists), even as those readers retain an awareness that the characters and events are invented. Imagine being at a powerful performance of Shakespeare's *Othello*. In Act V, as Othello is about to strangle Desdemona, you will feel pity and fear as you simultaneously strongly desire that Othello won't follow through on his plan and fully expect that he will. As you feel these emotions, you will stay in your seat to watch what happens rather than running onto the stage to stop Othello. What's more, you're not a bad person for staying in your seat.

Your strong feelings arise from one part of your consciousness responding to Othello and Desdemona as if they were real, while your decision to stay in your seat arises from another part of your consciousness knowing that they are not real but invented. Rhetorical theorists call the first part of your consciousness the narrative audience, and the second part the authorial audience. Furthermore, they explain that you're not a bad person by noting that the narrative audience position (the "as if" position) is nested within the authorial audience position (the "they are" position). Going further, rhetorical theorists identify the narrative audience position as that of an observer within the fiction, a place from which readers can see without being seen. I have suggested adapting J.K. Rowling's invention of the Invisibility Cloak as a metaphor to help explain the activity of the rhetorical reader joining the narrative audience (Phelan, 2018). That reader dons an Invisibility Cloak and steps into the world of the fiction, and under that Cloak, they can observe the characters and events without being observed.

As Peter J. Rabinowitz, the rhetorical theorist who first proposed the distinction between the authorial and narrative audiences, has explained (1998), the greater the overlap between the knowledge and beliefs of the narrative and authorial audiences, the greater the degree of realism in the fiction. In "The Yellow Wallpaper," the only significant difference is that the narrative audience regards the characters and events as actual, while the authorial audience knows that they are invented. By contrast, the authorial and narrative audiences of J.K. Rowling's Harry Potter novels diverge in their beliefs about magic, Invisibility Cloaks, fantastic creatures, and many other things.

More generally, then, in "The Yellow Wallpaper," rhetorical readers simultaneously respond to Gilman's character narrator as a real person and retain the tacit knowledge that she is invented. In the narrative audience, they feel a great deal of sympathy and distress for her as her perceptions of the wallpaper in the room to which she is confined become increasingly distorted. Since the authorial audience remains aware that Gilman has invented this character narrator, they also become interested in Gilman's purposes.

In "This Old Man," by contrast, there is no narrative audience, because the character Roger Angell is not invented but real. Actual readers do not need an Invisibility Cloak to enter his world because they are already part of it. At the same time, rhetorical readers recognize that Angell the writer and Angell the character are not identical. Instead, Angell the writer offers one representation of himself focusing on his age. That representation does not depend on Angell's inventing either himself or events but rather on selecting and emphasizing aspects of his character, his life, and his current condition. Thus, both Gilman and Angell actively construct their characters, but Gilman's construction involves the shaping of invented materials while Angell's involves a shaping of the actual.

This distinction in nonfictional first-person narrative between the author and the character (or experiencing-I) is even clearer in Tobias Wolff's retrospective memoir, *In Pharaoh's Army*. The occasion of Wolff's telling is in 1994, 25 years after the main events he narrates. This temporal distance facilitates his clear-eyed and often self-critical view of who-he-was-then. Even when Wolff is not especially self-critical, rhetorical readers will note his shifts from his perspective at the time of the action (that is, the perspective of the experiencing-I) to his perspective at the time of the telling (that of the narrating-I). For example, in "Close Calls," he introduces his account of his second brush with death this way: "My second close call was of a more civilian character, the kind of thing that happens on road crews and construction sites. Still, it almost nailed me" (91). The "me" is of course continuous with the Wolff who is constructing this telling, but rhetorical readers register that the "me" is not identical with that constructor. Instead, the "me" is Wolff the character who almost died and whose experience Wolff the author is narrating. I'll have more to say about how rhetorical readers negotiate Wolff's handing of the teller–character relationships in my detailed analysis of "Close Calls" in Chapter 10. I'll also discuss perspectival shifts in more detail in Chapter 5.

As the discussion so far indicates, the narrative and authorial audiences are positions that actual rhetorical readers take on. In addition, just as narratives typically have a narrator, that narrator typically has an audience, called a narratee. Authors vary widely in the degrees to which they characterize their narratees and in the kinds of relations they establish between narratees and the authorial and narrative audiences. In some fictional narratives, such as Colm Tóibín's "One Minus One," which I'll discuss in Chapter 4, a character narrator will address another character, and, thus, the narratee will be clearly distinct from both the narrative and authorial audiences. In other realist fictions, such as "The Yellow Wallpaper," the narratee will be only minimally characterized and the narrator's address to that narratee functions as direct communication to the narrative audience. Furthermore, in "The Yellow Wallpaper," the only significant difference between the narratee and the narrative audience, on the one hand, and the authorial audience, on the other, is that the first two are located in the storyworld and the third is not.

In nonfiction narratives, authors typically want the authorial audience and the narratee to coincide, though if I were to write "An Open Letter to President Joe Biden," I could take advantage of the difference between my narratee and my authorial audience. In "This Old Man," Angell's narratee and authorial audience coincide so that when he moves to implicit direct address as in phrases such as "Never mind," he is talking directly to his authorial audience.

Now just as authors can have in mind an ideal target audience, so too can narrators. Authors can then take advantage of differences between ideal and actual narratees by showing how narrators adjust their telling when they recognize that their actual addressees are not responding as they had intended. In such cases rhetorical readers (in their authorial and narrative audience positions) will find the narrator–narratee relationship an additional source of narrative interest. That is, rhetorical readers will be interested not only in the told of the narrative (the characters and events) but also in the telling. Joyce Carol Oates in "Hospice/Honeymoon," a story we will consider in Chapter 5, gets a lot of mileage from the discrepancy between ideal and actual narratees.

Question 2. In giving so much weight to reading in the authorial audience, does rhetorical reading risk claiming too much certainty about authors' intentions? Does it seek to impose a standard of "one right reading" that is both epistemologically and ethically untenable?

The short answer is no. Answering yes would mean denying what it's like to be a rhetorical reader, especially the experiences of learning from other readers, whether that learning involves a recognition of erroneous interpretation or of how others' interpretations offer more powerful accounts of the connections between readerly experiences and their sources in the teller's construction of the narrative.

The longer answer is also no, and it involves articulating some additional principles about reading and then discussing how they relate to the possibility and desirability of actual audiences becoming members of an authorial audience.

Principle 1. Authors want to be understood by their target audiences. This principle underlies our treatment of just about all non-literary communication, and, indeed, of nonfictional literary communication. Even in cases in which a speaker seeks to foil all efforts at understanding, the force of their resistance derives in part from the default assumption. Rhetorical theory extends this assumption to literary communication: authors are motivated to write because they have things they want to share with others, and many readers read because they want to know and to learn from what authors have to share. Furthermore, while authors of literary narrative often have broader audiences than speakers in oral conversation, those authors inevitably presuppose things about what those audiences know, believe, value, and so on. Close reading can yield productive hypotheses about those presuppositions and the purposes that they're part of.

Most readers will applaud an effort to determine what Angell wants to communicate about old age in "This Old Man," but many readers trained in literary theory will be less enthusiastic about a corresponding effort to determine (in the sense of pin down) what Gilman wants to communicate about her subject matter. The reasons for this lack of enthusiasm are many, but I'll single out here the legacies of the New Criticism with its labeling of reading for authorial purposes the "Intentional Fallacy" and of post-structuralism with its proclamation of the "Death of the Author." Rhetorical theory questions the idea that the distinction between fiction and nonfiction should be so consequential for the effort to understand authorial communication. In both cases we have authors using language and other resources to achieve certain purposes in relation to target audiences. Rhetorical theory acknowledges that Gilman's communication, with her use of an unreliable narrator whose unreliability increases as the story progresses, is less straightforward than Angell's. But rhetorical theory does not find that these differences warrant the conclusion that actual readers can join Angell's authorial audience but not Gilman's. Instead, it finds that Gilman's strategies are motivated by her interest in capturing for her authorial audience the complexities and nuances of her character narrator's experiences.

Principle 2. Entering the authorial audience is often a way for a reader to add to their store of experiences, to increase their knowledge about the world, to challenge their beliefs and values, and to accrue other benefits. In other words, the assumption is that moving as much as possible from the prison-house of one's own subjectivity into the perspective of another person has the potential to enhance one's life. (Whether that potential is realized depends of course not just on the success of the effort but also on the quality of the other's perspective.) The young person who enters into Angell's communication about what it's like to be a 93-year-old man can increase their understanding of the life course and perhaps change their attitudes about the elderly. The twenty-first century male chauvinist who enters into Gilman's audience and takes on the character narrator's and Gilman's perspective may undergo a conversion experience.

These examples also indicate that different actual readers are likely to find some authorial audiences easier to enter than others. Readers closer to Angell's age are likely to be more primed to enter his audience than readers in their teens and 20s. Women who've suffered as a consequence of the attitudes of apparently well-meaning patriarchal male doctors are more likely to ease into Gilman's audience than those doctors are. I stopped teaching Leo Tolstoy's "The Death of Ivan Ilych" a few years ago because I found that young twenty-first century American students had a lot of trouble entering into Tolstoy's authorial audience. Tolstoy invites that audience to share Ivan's recognition of his mortality, but so many of my students either didn't see or didn't accept the invitation that the story fell flat for them.

Picking up on my parenthetical remark about the quality of the author's perspective, I add that rhetorical theory acknowledges that not all authorial audience positions are equal and that some, in fact, can be unhealthy to occupy. That's why rhetorical theory insists on the importance not only of understanding (via entering the authorial audience) but also of overstanding (assessing from one's position as actual reader the experience of being in the authorial audience).

Principle 3. Rhetorical readers regard their statements about the activities and interpretations of authorial audiences as hypotheses not definitive findings. This principle means that (a) rhetorical readers know that they are working with probabilities rather than certainties; and (b) their hypotheses are subject to testing against their own re-examinations of the feedback loop among authorial agency, textual phenomena, and readerly response and against competing hypotheses about that loop offered by other rhetorical readers.

In light of these principles, rhetorical readers offer their findings as invitations for further discussion rather than as statements that close it off. I therefore invite all readers of this book to disagree with my findings about the narratives I discuss and to propose new and better ones.

Question 3. Aren't there other valuable things to do in response to narratives than read them rhetorically?

The short answer is yes, praise the Lord. Rhetorical reading seeks one kind of valuable knowledge about narrative and its workings. Other modes of reading—historicist, structuralist, feminist, cognitive, sociolinguistic, and more—offer other kinds of valuable knowledge. My case for rhetorical reading, as I say in Chapter 1, is that it is flexible, multi-faceted, and coherent and that its focus on somebody telling somebody else is especially well-suited for the goals of Narrative Medicine. More than that, rhetorical theory's a posteriori stance toward interpretation means that it remains open to the insights of other approaches and is interested in integrating them into its understanding of authorial communication. This book offers multiple examples of this practice in subsequent chapters, and I'll note here that my brief discussion of "The Yellow Wallpaper" has been inflected by ideas from feminist narratology. Furthermore, ideas from other approaches can often inform the activity of overstanding. Again, though, rhetorical theory shies away from an eclecticism that would simply add up the insights offered by different approaches, preferring instead to develop interpretations that show how the multiple insights yield a viable larger account of the author-audience-purpose nexus.

Mimetic, Thematic, and Synthetic: Or Emotions, Ideas, Values, and Aesthetics

The rhetorical model of audiences also helps me identify and consider the functions of three broad components of narrative construction and readerly interest: the mimetic, the thematic, and the synthetic. These three components exist simultaneously and thus interact, but, for analytical purposes, we can distinguish among them. The mimetic is the source of our emotional responses, the thematic of our ideational responses, and the synthetic of our aesthetic ones. Here are working definitions:[1]

The mimetic component refers to the narrative's imitations of—or references to—the actual world including such matters as characters functioning as possible—or actual—people and events following the cause-effect logic of the extratextual world.

The thematic component refers to the ideational, ethical, and ideological dimensions of the narrative.

The synthetic component refers to narrative as itself a constructed object, something artificial rather than natural, something fashioned rather than found.

As noted earlier, these components are simultaneously present, but authors, depending on their purposes, may bring any one of them into the foreground or relegate any one into the background of their narrative constructions. In other words, in some narratives one of the three components will be most prominent, in others two will be prominent, and in still others all three will be prominent.

Angell uses his title "This Old Man" to direct his audience to focus on the mimetic and thematic components of his piece: not any old man or all old men, but this one (the mimetic); not everything about this man, but rather some particular things that are also shared by others, especially his age (the thematic). Furthermore, like many others, he sets up a mimetic-thematic feedback loop: the thicker the description of his individual situation the more material he has for thematizing it, and the more he offers generalizations of various kinds the more he illuminates his particular situation. To be sure, Angell invites his authorial audience to recognize that his piece is well-crafted (the synthetic), and of course actual audiences can make that craft their chief interest. But from the perspective of the authorial audience, Angell does not make the synthetic an equal (or even rival) interest. Instead, he uses it in the service of communicating his reflections on his condition at this stage of life. When we move to overstanding, the synthetic will often move into prominence, as indeed it would in my overstanding of Angell: how carefully and effectively he has constructed the piece (see my further discussion in Chapter 7 on Time).

Gilman's narrative sets up similar relationships among the three components, but its fictional status, which generates a narrative audience, adds another wrinkle. Since the narrative audience regards the character narrator and her experiences as real, the mimetic is prominent. But as the authorial audience reads for purpose, they recognize that the story sets up its mimetic-thematic feedback loop. The more the narrative and authorial audiences respond to the particulars of the character narrator's situation, the more the authorial audience recognizes her representative status. And the more they recognize Gilman's thematic points about patriarchal control, the deeper their sympathy with the character narrator as individual woman. Again, actual readers, when they move to overstanding, can step back and admire Gilman's synthetic construction of this relationship, especially through her handling of the increasingly unreliable narration. But, like Angell, Gilman uses her artful synthetic construction in the service of enhancing the story's mimetic and thematic effects. To put the point another way, Angell and Gilman use the synthetic to enhance the ways rhetorical readers feel and think deeply about the characters and situations.

Steps Two and Three of Rhetorical Reading: Overstanding and Springboarding

If understanding is about doing all one can to take on the perspectives of others—authors, narrators, and characters—overstanding and springboarding are about returning to one's own actual audience position and responding from it. As rhetorical readers engage in overstanding and springboarding, however, they will be open to revising their initial understandings. In other words, although the steps are analytically distinct, they frequently interact.

Overstanding

This last point sets up the first one I want to make about overstanding: it is not understanding's binary opposite but its dialogic partner. Understanding often goes hand-in-hand with appreciation and positive evaluation, as my discussions of Oates, Angell, and Gilman indicate. But it can also go hand-in-hand with negative judgments of the "don't go there" or "I can't believe the author just did that" variety. More than that, rhetorical reading views understanding and overstanding as dynamic, reciprocal activities. If, in doing the work of overstanding, I initially make a negative assessment of my reading experience, I can step back into my understanding with that assessment in mind. For example, I may have a negative response to a story such as Richard Selzer's "Imelda" because I think that it presupposes that white men are more important human beings than Brown women. But when I re-examine the story in order to substantiate my judgment, I may find that I have not been entirely fair to Selzer. But that re-examination and revision of my understanding may also lead me to consider other issues that provide the basis for a different negative evaluation. At that point, I can begin the process again. And so on.

Chapter 1 provides another example of such a dialogue in the discussion of "Widow's First Year." There, I revised my initial assessment that the story was flat and disappointing after reconsidering why Oates would run the risk of such a judgment and realizing that she was inviting her audience to pay attention to all that was implied in the widow's understatement. One might still assess the story as a poor representation of a widow's year of grief on the grounds that seven words are inevitably and hopelessly inadequate to capture that experience. And the dialogue could continue with the point that it's the very constraints of expression Oates puts on herself that makes the story effective.

As this example indicates, overstanding can involve both assessing the narrative on its own terms and assessing the terms themselves. If I say that Oates accomplishes a great deal with her seven words, then I'm saying that the story succeeds on its own terms. If I say that she could have done much better with a different seven words, then I'm saying that the story could work better on its own terms. (Aside: anyone who wants to push back on this overstanding can effectively do so by asking me to produce the more effective seven words.) If I say that Oates's seven words accomplish a great deal and then go on to say that what she accomplishes does not come close to capturing a widow's grief, I am saying that the story's terms are inadequate.

Just as understanding involves attending to the multiple layers of the narrative communication, overstanding can be directed toward any of those layers, or indeed any aspect of it. That is, overstanding may focus on the affective, ethical, cognitive, or aesthetic dimensions of the experience, especially as those dimensions intersect with the mimetic, thematic, and synthetic components of the narrative. For example, some readers may, upon reflection, decide that Gilman manipulates their emotions as she invites them to make overly simplistic ethical judgments of the character narrator and her husband. In this overstanding, the affective, the ethical, and the aesthetic dimensions of the experience interact.

This example also points to another significant difference between the activities of understanding and overstanding. With understanding, rhetorical reading seeks consensus about what entering the authorial audience entails.

(See the earlier discussion about interpretive hypotheses.) With overstanding and its return to the actual audience's positionality, rhetorical reading expects and welcomes different responses from different readers. Rhetorical readers can then discuss their differences, and as their overstandings lead them to reconsider their understandings, some may change their assessments. In this way, rhetorical readers can learn from each other. Sometimes, though, the discussion will end with readers agreeing to disagree. But that result too can be illuminating about the sources of the disagreement in the authorial construction of the text and about the subjectivity and positionality of the readers involved. In the next chapter, I'll consider a negative overstanding of "Imelda" and a response to it. But I do so with a recognition that the discussion I describe is just one of many that different groups of readers may have.

Springboarding

Both understanding and overstanding are activities tightly tethered to the author's narrative act and rhetorical readers' experiences with it. Their dialogic relationship emphasizes actual readers' interest in knowing the narrative act from the inside. Springboarding is what comes next, as rhetorical readers turn their attention outward toward the significance of the author's narrative act for their efforts to come to terms with the world and their places in it. Springboarding can take numerous forms. For example, a rhetorical reader may be inspired by their experiences to make a radical change in their behavior, or in a less radical way, may find a character who serves as a role model. Such readers make a habit of asking WWMRMD? (what would my role model do?). To take another example, a rhetorical reader may pick up on an idea in the narrative and run with it in some direction that never occurred to the author. As you think about how you respond to narratives, I'm sure you can think of other examples.

I want to highlight three other kinds of springboarding to further illustrate how it works. I choose these possibilities not only because they are common and important but also because they demonstrate an increasing movement away from the concerns of the author to those of the actual reader. These possibilities are (a) imaginative gap-filling; (b) unrestricted appropriating; and (c) creative rewriting.

Because narrative always involves selection and emphasis, it always contains gaps and thus leaves room for *imaginative gap-filling*. Oates's "Widow's First Year" is an especially clear example. Reading in the authorial audience we don't have sufficient warrants for specifying the challenges the widow faced in that year. But we can fill in the gaps with our own lists of challenges: she was beset by bouts of magical thinking; she lost her appetite; she abused drugs and alcohol; she suffered from depression. We can also invent lists of things she did to survive: she relied on the kindness of others; she read great literature; she wrote flash fiction. Such gap-filling not only takes Oates's story and expands it but also activates the actual reader's own imagination and allows them to find connections between the story and things they care about. To take just one more example: With "The Yellow Wallpaper," Gilman leaves a gap about whether John is a well-intentioned or ill-intentioned patriarch, and some rhetorical readers are likely to make a stronger connection between the narrative and their situations or understandings by choosing "well-intentioned," while others will make that connection by choosing "ill-intentioned." Still others may prefer to fill that gap first one way and then the other.

Unrestricted appropriating of a narrative involves rhetorical readers applying it to contexts and situations that are significantly different from those in which its author composed it, often ones that rhetorical readers find relevant to their own lives. Julius Caesar wrote "veni, vidi, vici" ("I came, I saw, I conquered") in 47 BC as a message to the Roman Senate to inform them about a quick victory in battle. But ever since students of history learned about Caesar's efficient narrative, they have used it to convey their own victories, regardless of their duration. This free appropriation also allows the teller to claim kin with Caesar's mastery. The huge gaps in Caesar's version make it easier to appropriate, but such gappiness is not a prerequisite for appropriation. Readers often appropriate parts of detailed narratives to make connections to their own experiences. "I am (or am not) a Pollyanna, a Hamlet, a Jay Gatsby." "I am a protagonist in a Thomas Hardy novel." "Like Lily Briscoe [in Virginia Woolf's *To the Lighthouse*], I have had my vision." To take another example, I might use "Widow's First Year" as a springboard to reflect on the hardest year of my life, or on a time when I expected to feel grief but didn't. Or I can read "The Yellow Wallpaper" and use it as a springboard to reflect on times when I was housebound, or when others didn't perceive things the way I did. And so on. The larger point is that my appropriation can move from the narrative in just about any direction.

Creative rewriting typically takes the form of another narrative that reshapes the materials of the original. The history of the novel includes a tradition of creative rewriting, with such notable examples as Henry Fielding's retelling of Samuel Richardson's *Pamela* in *Shamela*, Jean Rhys's retelling of Charlotte Brontë's *Jane Eyre* in *Wide Sargasso Sea*, and Peter Carey's retelling of Charles Dickens's *Great Expectations* in *Jack Maggs*. In these cases, the retellings are in dialogue with the original and they demonstrate both understanding and overstanding. Fan fiction is the most prominent contemporary example of creative rewriting. But the activity does not need to be either as elaborate or as ambitious as the novel-length rewritings or the extended fan fictions. Actual readers can do it in the privacy of their own Word programs, and their rewritings can be as simple or as elaborate as they find useful for their purposes.

Creative rewriting can take the form of adapting the premise of the narrative to a similar but related situation. I might, for example, read Angell's

"This Old Man" and think about how I would characterize myself as "This No Longer Middle-Aged Man." Someone else might think about how they would characterize themselves as "This Twenty-Something Woman." In such creative rewriting the reader need not follow the template of structure and topics in the original. Working with the premise is sufficient.

Again, as I go forward, I will focus primarily on understanding and then offer a few prompts to jumpstart the activities of overstanding and springboarding. But readers should feel free to engage in these activities according to their own particular interests.

Note

1 I develop these conceptions at greater length in a dialogue with Matthew Clark, who has a somewhat different take on each of the components. See *Debating Rhetorical Narratology*.

Works Cited

Angell, Roger. "This Old Man." *The New Yorker*, 9 February2014. www.new yorker.com/magazine/2014/02/17/old-man-3. (Accessed 13 December 2021).

Clark, Matthew and James Phelan. *Debating Rhetorical Narratology: On the Synthetic, Mimetic, and Thematic Aspects of Narrative.* Columbus, OH: Ohio State University Press, 2020. Open access at https://kb.osu.edu/handle/1811/90880

Gilman, Charlotte Perkins. "The Yellow Wallpaper." In *The Norton Anthology of Literature by Women: The Traditions in English*, 3rd ed., edited by Sandra M. Gilbert and Susan Gubar, 1392–1402. New York: W.W. Norton & Company, 2007 [1892].

Phelan, James. "Fictionality, Audiences, and Character: A Rhetorical Alternative to Catherine Gallagher's 'The Rise of Fictionality.'" *Poetics Today* 39, 1 (2018): 123–139.

Rabinowitz, Peter J. *Before Reading: Narrative Conventions and the Politics of Interpretation.* Columbus, OH: The Ohio State University Press, 1998 [1987].

3 Character and Progression I

Understanding and Overstanding Richard Selzer's "Imelda"

I pair these two resources in this chapter because, from the perspective of a reader's experience, they go hand-in-hand. I also devote the next chapter to different uses of these resources in order to underline both their significance and their diversity. Henry James famously expressed the co-dependence of character and plot (or, more precisely, event) this way: "What is character but the determination of incident? What is incident but the illustration of character?" (174). To come at the point somewhat differently, both progression and character are deeply intertwined with narrative's attention to change over time. Many narratives track a character (or a group of characters) who begin(s) in one position and end(s) up, as a result of their involvement in a series of events, in a significantly different one. This change of position often, though not always, is accompanied by a change in character. Indeed, genres such as the coming-of-age novel (aka the Bildungsroman) are organized around the representations of the intertwining of changes in character and changes in their positions. But even when the character remains unchanged, as in many detective novels where the protagonist serves as a site of stability in a dangerous world, the character's role in the overall trajectory of the narrative is an important focus of readerly interest. In addition, some stories switch the standard relationship between character and change over time, subordinating a mini-narrative to the dominant interest in revealing character. I call such stories portrait narratives and I will analyze one in the next chapter, Colm Tóibín's "One Minus One."

More generally, as I'll explain below, authors guide their audiences to be more interested in some components of character than others through their construction of the progression. By attending to both resources here, I can more fully support the claim I make in Chapter 1 about the payoffs of recognizing that authors shape their raw materials in some ways rather than others.

My procedure will be to offer a rhetorical account of these resources and then analyze how they are deployed in Richard Selzer's "Imelda," a narrative in which the central character's traits and position change over time. After the detailed analysis, rooted in an effort to understand the story on its own terms, I will sketch the contours of a debate about overstanding it. I will conclude with some general takeaways and some prompts for springboarding.

DOI: 10.4324/9781003018865-3

The initial rhetorical account of the resources involves the discussion of multiple terms and concepts in a short space, and I realize that the discussion offers a lot to take in all at once. But I'm hopeful that the concrete analyses will add clarity to that account and that, ultimately, you'll recognize a benefit in having the theoretical account all in one place. To aid a first reading, I have put key points in **bold**.

Progression and Plot

Progression subsumes plot. Narrative theorists agree that plot is the interrelated sequence of events in a narrative, but they disagree about its overall importance to narrative relative to other elements such as character. Most of us are familiar with the attitude that "reading for the plot" is an unsophisticated way to engage with narrative because it keeps readers' attention on the allegedly superficial level of what-happens-next. For theorists who subscribe to this view, plot is a necessary part of narrative (indeed, for some, an almost necessary evil) but not the primary source of its power. Such theorists often regard character as more important than plot, as E.M. Forster argues in his influential *Aspects of the Novel* (1927).

Other theorists, by contrast, see plot as central to narrative construction and narrative experience, and, thus, more important than character. In the *Poetics*, for example, Aristotle famously claims that plot is the most significant element of tragedy. Peter Brooks uses the full title of his book to express his view of the resource's importance: *Reading for the Plot: Design and Intention in Narrative*. Aristotle, Brooks, and other theorists who take the plot-is-central position contend that plot is the main mechanism for organizing a narrative. Plot organizes a narrative's multiple characters and events into an intelligible whole. In this way, plot is crucial to narrative as a way of knowing.

By subsuming plot under progression, rhetorical theory, in one sense, side-steps this debate, and, in another, resolves it. Rhetorical theory's move sidesteps the debate by saying that some narratives make plot central and some make character—or some other resource—central. The move resolves the debate by saying that progression is more important than either plot or character. More generally, **the concept of progression follows from the principles that narrative as a rhetorical action is itself a dynamic event that unfolds in time and that understanding the principles underlying that movement can take us a long way toward grasping a narrative's purposes.**

More specifically, progression is a synthesis of two kinds of movement, what I call textual dynamics and readerly dynamics. Developments in the textual movement of narrative generate a trajectory of responses in audiences, even as an author's awareness of their audiences influences their construction of the textual dynamics. For example, an author interested in surprising their audience will be careful to construct the textual dynamics so that they do not spoil the surprise even as they contain covert clues about it.

Subsuming plot under progression also enables the recognition that textual dynamics is itself a synthesis of two other components: plot dynamics (the mechanism underlying the relation of events to each other) and narratorial dynamics (the mechanisms underlying the telling of those events). Narratives with unreliable narrators highlight the importance of narratorial dynamics: following the trajectory of the narrative entails attending to both what happens and how the teller represents it. I'll say more about unreliability in Chapter 5 on "Tellers," but since Selzer uses this resource, I'll just sketch my approach here. **Authors use narrators to do three main things—report, interpret what they report, and evaluate it. When authors endorse their performances, the narration is reliable. When authors signal that they do not endorse their narrators' reports, interpretations, or evaluations, the narration is unreliable.** Narrators can be partially reliable and partially unreliable, as often happens when they report reliably but interpret and evaluate unreliably. Selzer's and Tóibín's narrators function this way.

Finally, **subsuming plot under progression allows us to recognize that narrative lends itself to hybrid forms, including portrait narrative, lyric narrative, and essay narrative.** In these forms, progression remains crucial, while plot plays a subordinate role. In portrait narrative, as mentioned above, plot is subordinated to the unfolding revelation of a character. In portrait narrative, event sequences contribute backstory, functioning primarily as further illustration of the character. In "My Last Duchess," for example, Robert Browning reveals the Duke of Ferrara's character through the Duke's monologue about his art collection, addressed to a representative from the unnamed Count who is the father of his soon-to-be next duchess. That monologue includes backstory—he tells the representative what happened to the previous duchess (he had her put to death for smiling too freely)—and both that story and his audacity to tell it on this occasion to this audience reveal who he is: an egotistical, imperious, possessive man who wants everyone to recognize they should defer to his wishes without his ever having to make them explicit. He did not speak directly to his duchess because doing so would entail "some stooping" and "I choose never to stoop." His aversion to stooping also means that he uses his overt conversation about his art collection to send the covert but clear message about how he wants the next duchess to behave. The Duke's monologue begins "That's my last duchess painted on the wall." Browning implicitly says "This is my Duke of Ferrara painted on the page." Tóibín's "One Minus One," as I'll discuss in the next chapter, also uses a speaker's monologue as the basis of a portrait narrative.

In lyric narrative, plot is subordinated to the unfolding revelation of a particular situation, especially of a character in a situation. In lyric narrative, then, situation is more important than character, whereas in portrait narrative character is more important than situation. In the lyric hybrid, the event sequences of plot either contribute relevant backstory or help reveal aspects of the character's situation, even as the text is organized around exploring the salient dimensions of that situation. In the short story "Barbie-Q," for example, Sandra Cisneros presents a lower-class young Latina character narrator whose situation does not change. Instead, Cisneros devotes the story to exploring the nature of that situation and how the character narrator deals with it. In the last paragraph, she insists that the Barbie dolls she and her sister recently acquired at a fire sale on Maxwell Street in Chicago (the backstory) are as good as, say, the unsullied ones purchased at full price by white girls in the suburbs. Cisneros indicates that her character narrator protests too much, but she also invites her readers to recognize this desire about the dolls stands in for the character narrator's larger desire for equality. Her expression of that desire in this way reveals a lot about both her situation and her way of dealing with it. Roger Angell's "This Old Man," which I'll discuss briefly in Chapter 6 on Perspective and Voice and more fully in Chapter 7 on Time, is a nonfictional lyric narrative devoted to capturing his situation as a 93-year-old man.

In essay narrative, plot is juxtaposed with a teller's multiple reflections on something, their identification of problems and proposing of solutions, or their making arguments. That is, the author of an essay narrative designs the event sequences and these essay-features to be mutually illuminating; the essay-features may even be ultimately in service of the event sequences. Damon Tweedy's *Black Man in a White Coat*, a work that I'll discuss in Chapter 5 on "Tellers," is constructed as a series of essay narratives. Jesmyn Ward's "On Witness and Respair," the piece I use in my sketch of a Rhetorical Narrative Medicine workshop in Chapter 11 is another example of an essay narrative. Essay narratives are typically nonfictional.

The discussion of these hybrid forms—portrait narrative, lyric narrative, and essay narrative—invites a look, first, at poetry and, second, at argument, and their capacity for serving the purposes of Narrative Medicine. Although we commonly associate narrative and essay with prose and lyric with poetry, rhetorical theory views all three as modes of expression independent of whether the author writes all the way to the right-hand margin. In other words, some poetry is lyric (Robert Frost's "Nothing Gold Can Stay"), some is narrative (the *Iliad*), and some is the hybrid form lyric narrative (Frost's "Home Burial").[1] In addition, some is portrait narrative ("My Last Duchess") and some essay narrative (Frost's "Design"). And the same goes for prose. Narrative poetry, lyric poetry, and poetic hybrids as well as portrait narratives and essay narratives about medical and health issues can all serve the purposes of Narrative Medicine because all can offer valuable insights into those issues (contributing to our knowing-that) even as the work of understanding them can improve readers' skills in listening, perspective-taking, and empathizing (contributing to knowing-how).

Before going deeper into different ways authors synthesize textual and readerly dynamics, I find it helpful to bring character into the discussion.

Character as Mimetic, Thematic, and Synthetic

In *Aspects of the Novel*, E.M. Forster famously identified two kinds of character: round and flat. Round characters are capable of surprising readers in a plausible manner, while flat characters can be summed up by one or two unchanging traits. Forster's distinction is helpful as a rough-and-ready classification—and for that reason, it remains influential—but rhetorical theory seeks to go beyond its binary thinking and offer an account that does better justice to the complexity of the resource. The rhetorical account focuses less on types and plausible surprises and more on three components of the authorial construction of and readerly interest in narrative. In Chapter 1, I defined these three components and noted that they apply more specifically to character. Here are the general definitions and then the adaptations of them for character:

The mimetic component refers to the narrative's imitations of—or references to—the actual world including such matters as characters functioning as possible—or actual—people and events following the cause-effect logic of the extratextual world.

The thematic component refers to the ideational, ethical, and ideological dimensions of the narrative.

The synthetic component refers to narrative as itself a constructed object—something artificial rather than natural, something fashioned rather than found.

The mimetic component of character refers to **its function as a representation of a possible person**. To be sure, some narratives feature non-human characters or human characters with superpowers, but all such characters have at least one trait of a possible person. Furthermore, some characters are more fully developed representations of possible people than others. Forster, in effect, proposes that there are two main mimetic categories of character. Authors develop mimetic characters by assigning them multiple traits, including identity markers, and individuating characteristics (physical or mental attributes, habits of thought or behavior, including ways of responding to situations and interacting with others). Authors can then give emphasis to some traits, while leaving others in the background.

The thematic component of character refers to **its representative and/or ideational function**. The readerly habit of discerning an author's views about classes of people from their depiction of individual characters (what does William Shakespeare's depiction of Shylock in *The Merchant of Venice* reveal about his attitudes toward the Jews?) points to the presence and significance of the thematic function. Thus, a character with any culturally marked identity feature—gender, sexuality, race, disability, illnesses of various kinds, and so on—can represent larger groups who share that identity, and, by extension, can represent certain larger groups who share an intersectional identity. Some authors will thematize some identity markers and not others, and such decisions can be revealing about what authors take for granted and what they expect their audiences to. For example, some narratives make whiteness the default racial identity of their characters, while others call attention to whiteness as a marked feature. And the same holds for other identity markers. How authors handle the marking and thematizing of identity features is often a rich issue to explore in overstanding, as we'll see with "Imelda."

In addition, sometimes characters represent ideas or abstract concepts. This ideational function is especially clear in allegories that rely on a one-to-one correspondence between a character and a concept.

The synthetic component of character refers to **its function in the larger design of the narrative.** Referring to a character as a protagonist or antagonist is invoking their synthetic function. Henry James talked about the "ficelle" character, one whose interactions with the protagonist allowed James to disclose to his readers in a plausible fashion important information about the protagonist and their situation. The "ficelle" is a character whose mimetic function is subordinated to their synthetic function. More generally, whenever we describe characters with such expressions as "X is the life force in this story" or "Y is the foil for the protagonist," we are also tapping into the synthetic function.

Any representation of character will simultaneously activate all three components, though different narratives can make one, two, or all three the main focus of readerly interest. In nonfiction narrative and realist fictions in print authors typically foreground the mimetic and thematic components and background the synthetic. In graphic narrative, as I'll discuss in Chapter 9, the synthetic is typically one of the foregrounded components. Regardless of the medium, the synthetic is always present, and readers can easily bring it into the foreground, if they're so inclined.

Since progression is the mechanism by which a narrative guides its audience's interests in one, two, or all three components, I now turn to a more detailed look at how it works in standard (that is, non-hybrid) narrative.

Progression: Plot Dynamics, Narratorial Dynamics, and Readerly Dynamics

Plot dynamics and narratorial dynamics are, in a sense, a narrative's motor, the forces that set and sustain it in motion until it reaches its destination. Key to their workings are instabilities (for plot dynamics) and tensions (for narratorial dynamics). Instabilities refer to unsettled situations between or among characters or between a character and their situation, while tensions refer to unsettled relations between or among authors, narrators, and audiences. Unreliable narration, for example, introduces tensions into the progression. So too does narration in which the teller points to the differences between what they know and what their narratee knows. **Instabilities and tensions often interact in ways that deepen audiences' engagement with a narrative's progression.**

Plot's forward movement typically begins with the disruption of one or more characters' state(s) of equilibrium, or with an event that takes one or more characters dealing with an existing unstable state in a new direction. This disruption often functions as the global instability of the narrative. This forward movement is typically framed by some kind of exposition about character, space, time, and other relevant contextual information. This exposition can also be distributed across the progression, depending on the teller's judgments about the relative efficacy of disclosing information sooner or later.

Jane Austen's *Pride and Prejudice,* with the arrival of the single man of good fortune into the Longbourn neighborhood, is a good example of a sudden disruption, while Homer's *Iliad,* with Achilles's wrath during the already disruptive Trojan War, is a strong example of the second kind. Plot typically continues through its middle by tracing how the initial instability leads to various complications, as the characters' efforts to deal with it lead to further disruptions or bring in some other unanticipated problems. Plot typically moves to its end when the potential within the complications for some new, satisfactory direction gets realized. This move toward resolution may be the result of the characters' efforts and the ways they've changed, those of other forces (such as the whims of Fortune), or some combination of the two. **We can capture the temporal movement of plot dynamics with the metaphor of a journey, consisting of launch (beginning)—voyage (middle)—arrival (ending).**

Narratorial dynamics refer to the relationships among tellers and their audiences across beginning, middle, and ending. Sometimes authors, narrators, and audiences align, and sometimes they don't. When they don't, we have tensions. We can get at narratorial dynamics by asking questions about such matters as reliability, tone, and decisions about what to disclose when. Furthermore, the answers to these questions can change as we move from beginning through middle to end. **We can capture the temporal movement of narratorial dynamics with the metaphor of a relationship, consisting of initiation (beginning), interaction (middle), and farewell (ending).**

Readerly dynamics, as noted above, both follow from and influence textual dynamics. Readerly dynamics include multiple layers of interacting responses: inferencing (at the cognitive level), feeling (the affective level), and judging (the ethical level). The responses interact in a feedback loop as cognitive interpretations influence ethical judgments, and those judgments influence affective responses—and as affect influences ethics and ethics influences cognition. We can capture the temporal movement of readerly dynamics with the metaphor of discovery-over-time and the reminder that ethical judgments and emotional responses accompany that discovery. **The shorthand description of that discovery process is the sequence: initial configuration of the narrative and its likely shape (beginning), intermediate (re)configuration (middle), and final (re)configuration (ending).**

Understanding Narrative Progression and Character in Richard Selzer's "Imelda"

Richard Selzer's "Imelda" is a remarkable story about a brilliant American plastic surgeon, Hugh Franciscus, told by one of his former students, about how Franciscus's encounter with two Honduran women, the young Imelda and her mother, changed him irrevocably. This description does not say much about either the progression or the purposes of the story, but rather begins to identify its raw materials. I start my analysis this way in order to link rhetorical theory's idea that a teller shapes their materials (the basic "story stuff") in some ways rather than others with the importance rhetorical theory gives to progression. In identifying the raw materials, I do not claim to know details about Selzer's process of composing the story. Instead, I'm making an analytical claim for heuristic purposes: recognizing that Selzer builds the story out of these materials can yield substantial insight into how he constructs the progression to achieve his larger purposes.

Applying this heuristic procedure to "Imelda," I find three central characters and four key events. The characters are Franciscus, Imelda, and her mother. I'll explain shortly why I do not see the character narrator as one of the key fundamental materials of the story but instead as a crucial invention for Selzer's treatment of that material. The events are Franciscus's first meeting with Imelda; Imelda's dying on the operating table as Franciscus gets ready to repair her cleft lip and palate; her mother's expressing gratitude that Franciscus has fixed her daughter's appearance before she meets her Maker; and Franciscus then doing the operation in the morgue.

In what follows I offer a detailed analysis of Selzer's shaping of these materials, but here's the big picture:

1   Selzer uses these characters and events as the main resources for his telling a story of Franciscus's ethical decisions in relation to Imelda and how those decisions altered his character.
2   Selzer invents the character narrator and the ensuing narratorial dynamics to put Franciscus's mimetic traits into sharp relief and to heighten the stakes of his ethical decisions. More particularly, Selzer uses the character narrator's initial unreliable evaluation of Franciscus's decision to operate on Imelda's corpse and his final reliable evaluation of that decision to introduce and then resolve a key tension in the narrative.
3   Selzer uses a determinate ambiguity at the end of the plot dynamics to further deepen rhetorical readers' affective and ethical engagement with the progression.

Now on to the more detailed analysis. We can begin, as I noted in Chapter 1, by attending to the feedback loop among authorial agency, textual phenomena, and readerly response. Since we can pick any point in the loop, I choose readerly response, giving special attention to the intertwining of its affective and ethical dimensions. I'm gripped by the sequence of Franciscus's interactions with Imelda and her mother and especially by his unexpected decision to operate on Imelda after her death. That sequence—and my own ethical judgments about it—result in a powerful mixture of emotional responses: empathy/sympathy, sorrow for all three characters, approbation of Imelda's mother and Franciscus in their meeting after Imelda's death, ethical and affective uncertainty about his decision to operate. (I also begin to overstand the story during this sequence, something I'll address later.) These readerly responses, then, lead me to the hypothesis that Selzer's purposes are to move his audience emotionally by means of engaging them with the characters and the thematic and ethical issues in that sequence. More specifically, he uses that engagement to advance a case for the power of human connection in medical interactions and for the resulting complexity of ethical decision-making about many aspects of such interactions.

This hypothesis can guide an analysis of his construction of the progression, even as that analysis can lead to further development of the hypothesis. My readerly response and this hypothesis make visible several features of his shaping of his raw materials into the completed progression.

1   Selzer delays introducing the global instability—Imelda's death—until just after the halfway point of the story. The first half is given over to exposition and to establishing a secondary track of the progression concerned with the relation between Franciscus and the character narrator (see #4 below).

2   Selzer shows that the ensuing complications are easily resolved at the level of action—Franciscus tells Imelda's mother; she forgives him; he operates; she is pleased with the result—but he uses the narratorial dynamics to add significant layers of affective and ethical complexity to that sequence, complexity that means the overall progression does not resolve until later.

3   Selzer magnifies the importance of Franciscus's post-mortem operation by using his character narrator to pass a negative ethical judgment on it and then to reconstruct the scene in his imagination. (Although Selzer does not explicitly identify the character narrator's gender, I will use "he, him, his" pronouns, because I believe that for Selzer, as he was writing in the 1970s, the unmarked gender was masculine, and that during the time of the action, which is many years before the time of the telling, the great majority of medical students were men. A similar logic applies to my interpreting both Franciscus and the character narrator as white.)

4   Selzer uses the secondary track of the progression to bring the story to its resolution. This resolution has two parts. The main track and this secondary track converge when Franciscus makes a presentation to his colleagues and students about the trip to Comayagua, Honduras, and the character narrator realizes that Franciscus is on the verge of showing

them a photograph of his operation on Imelda. The character narrator intervenes and thus keeps Franciscus from exposing what everyone in his audience would regard as a violation of medical ethics.

5   In the second step toward resolution, Selzer moves from scene to summary—the character narrator covers more than 15 years in a single paragraph—and then has the character narrator offer a final reflection from his perspective at the time of the telling.

Each of these features deserves additional commentary.

1 The Deferred Launch: Franciscus's Character and the Profile of the Character Narrator

Three aspects of Selzer's construction here stand out: (a) the initiation into the narratorial dynamics; (b) the mimetic portrait of Franciscus; and (c) the secondary track of the progression.

With regard to the narratorial dynamics, Selzer makes three key choices: as noted above, he makes the character narrator a former student of Franciscus and designates the time of narration as many years after the main events—indeed, it's the death of his former teacher that prompts the character narrator's telling. He also gives the character narrator a limited but significant relationship with Franciscus that develops to some degree over the course of the action. By making the character narrator Franciscus's former student, Selzer can efficiently indicate the notable effects Franciscus had on others. By locating the telling many years after the main action, Selzer gives the character narrator the advantages of retrospection and reflection, thus enhancing his reliability when he narrates from his perspective at the time of the telling. The temporal distance enables the character narrator to see the events at the time of the action more clearly, to accurately trace their main consequences, and to comment insightfully on their significance. In these ways, Selzer constructs the initiation so that he puts his audience in the hands of a friendly, trustworthy guide to the story about Franciscus.

Furthermore, Selzer's choice of the time of the telling doesn't preclude his shifting to the character narrator's perspective at the time of the action. As Selzer takes advantage of that flexibility for the narration of (some of) the key events, he typically makes the character narrator a reliable on-the-scene reporter of those events, but he also creates the potential for him, given his youth and inexperience, to be an unreliable interpreter or evaluator of them. In addition, by choosing a character narrator, Selzer necessarily limits his access to Franciscus's interiority. Selzer turns this limitation into a positive feature when he uses it to introduce the significant ambiguity in the first part of the resolution. Finally, by choosing an observer character narrator, Selzer almost automatically establishes the second track of the progression.

This analysis of Selzer's choices sheds further light on the relationships among raw materials, shaping, and purposes. More particularly, it suggests that the character narrator is not part of the basic story stuff but rather a consequence of what Selzer wants to do with that stuff. In other words, Selzer's choices about the character narrator and his narration are motivated less by a primary interest in that character narrator and more by the functions Selzer needs him to perform. This analysis also illuminates the relationship among the character narrator's mimetic, thematic, and synthetic components: mimetically he's a perceptive and reflective former student; thematically, he's a representative of a younger generation that looks up to Franciscus; and synthetically, he functions as a device to regulate readerly access to Franciscus and to show his effect on others.

Selzer's handling of the narratorial dynamics feeds into his initial handling of the plot dynamics. The character narrator's comment on the occasion of the telling (he's just heard about the death of Franciscus) provides the motivation for the exposition, devoted to a sketch of the mimetic component of Franciscus's character. Franciscus is a dedicated, brilliant plastic surgeon, one who has mastered both its science and art. He is called arrogant by his enemies, he is a "zealous hunter," and he is rumored to be a ladies' man. The character narrator and his fellow students view Franciscus as "heroic, someone made up of several gods" (84). The character narrator notes that Franciscus has no close friends and that he is forthright but business-like with all his patients. Franciscus delivers to them all the relevant information and gives "good news and bad with the same dispassion" (84). In short, Franciscus's mimetic portrait readily links to his thematic component: he is one version of the masculine Type A personality: hard-driving at work and at play, the best at what he does, yet lacking in empathy for his patients and not capable of forming any strong interpersonal relationships. This exposition activates Selzer's audience interest in Franciscus and what will happen to him even as it does not clearly guide the audience's expectations. At this point, Selzer's readers bond more with the character narrator than with Franciscus.

After the exposition, Selzer uses a short sequence of local instability—minor complication—quick resolution to add to the sketch of the character narrator's mimetic component and to launch the second track of the progression. The character narrator describes himself as a typical third-year student: he lacks confidence in his skills and is terrified of doing the wrong thing as he begins working on the hospital wards. But his behavior during his observation of Franciscus doing a skin graft procedure begins to differentiate him. When the patient begins to speak rapidly in Spanish, Franciscus asks if anyone can translate, and the character narrator jumps right in, enabling Franciscus to relieve the patient's pain. Selzer uses the incident to reveal what the character narrator will not explicitly say about himself: he possesses good judgment and the confidence to act upon that judgment. This revelation adds to the affective and ethical bond between the character narrator and Selzer's audience as the narratorial dynamics move from initiation to interaction. Rhetorical readers' guide in the narrative is far more other-directed than self-interested.

The incident launches the second track of the progression because it establishes a relationship between the character narrator and Franciscus. The incident prompts Franciscus to invite the character narrator to serve as the translator and photographer during Franciscus's upcoming trip to Honduras. With the announcement of the trip, rhetorical readers make an initial configuration that the story will be about Franciscus's remarkable exploits on the trip, exploits that will further reveal his character and secondarily involve the character narrator.

During the first part of the trip, Franciscus and the character narrator relate as teacher-student/boss-employee, as they cope with the heat and provide care to many patients. The character narrator notes that Franciscus maintains his usual dispassionate approach to his patients and even to him. Despite their spending so much time together, "there were no overtures of friendship from Dr. Franciscus. He knew my place, and I knew it too" (87). With this move on the mimetic level, Selzer gives greater guidance to his audience's ethical judgments of Franciscus. His commitment to the social hierarchy of power and authority interferes with his ability to make a strong human connection, even in this situation where the two rely so much on each other. Selzer reinforces his audience's judgments that Franciscus is an admirable surgeon but a limited human being. At the same time, Selzer uses these developments on the mimetic level to simultaneously make the synthetic move of keeping the character narrator in the observer role.

2 The Launch and First Stage of the Voyage: The Characters of Imelda and Her Mother; Franciscus's Character Revisited

First, it's notable that, as Honduran women, Imelda and her mother are different from Franciscus in gender, race, class, and religion, and these differences loom large in the interactions between them. (Selzer's handling of these differences will be part of my overstanding later.) Imelda's mimetic character is defined by her Honduran identity, her age, the severity of her cleft lip and palate, and her way of handling her condition: she resists showing it to Franciscus. The character narrator notes that both her appearance and her resistance lead Franciscus to regard her as an extraordinary patient: "Had she brought her mouth to him willingly without shame, she would have been for him neither more nor less than any other patient" (89). Instead, Franciscus "must have been awed by the sight" of her, and the character narrator notes that the awe "flit[s] across his face for an instant" (89).

Despite—or perhaps because of—his awe at Imelda and her condition, Franciscus again demonstrates his mastery of the art and science of his specialty by developing a viable plan for corrective surgery. Yet, as Franciscus begins to execute the plan, the anesthesiologist stops him because Imelda has an allergic reaction that quickly becomes full-blown malignant hyperthermia and leads to her death. This moment, fully dramatized by the dialogue, constitutes the launch. The extraordinary doctor loses his extraordinary patient, one who has moved him, however briefly, beyond his dispassionate attitude. How will he respond?

His first response combines his professionalism with a new effort at human connection. He goes to Imelda's mother, and, rather than having the character narrator translate, he speaks to her directly, doing the best he can with his halting Spanish. And while he maintains his professionalism, his dispassion has vanished. He can barely move his lips, his voice is dry and dusty, he cannot keep the corner of his mouth from twitching. After Imelda's mother utters the word, "'Muerte,'" and he replies, "'Si, muerte,'" the character narrator notes that "he was like someone cast, still alive, as an effigy for his own tomb" (92). He closes his eyes and keeps them closed until the woman puts her hand on his arm, "a touch from which he did not withdraw" (92). The two stand silently gazing at each other and registering each other's grief. Finally, the woman gathers herself, tells Franciscus not to be sad because God's will has been done. And she is "happy" that her daughter will go to Heaven without her cleft lip. Franciscus does not tell her that Imelda died before he could do the surgery.

Selzer designs this sequence to radically alter rhetorical readers' responses to Franciscus. By depicting his ethically responsible actions, his grief for Imelda, his human connection with the mother, all of which exceed anything that he has ever had with a patient or a member of the patient's family, Selzer seeks to generate both admiration and empathy for Franciscus.

At the same time, the unfolding of the scene creates another significant complication of the plot dynamics in Franciscus's failure to correct Imelda's mother's belief that he has performed the operation. Is this an ethical failure? What will happen when she returns with her sons to retrieve Imelda's body the next day? Rhetorical readers' intermediate configuration revises the initial one: while the story is still about Franciscus's remarkable exploits, it is now about how he copes with unanticipated failure and the complications created by the miscommunications about it. At this point in the progression, Selzer does not offer his readers assurances about the outcome.

3 The Post-Mortem Operation: Complications in the Voyage and Narratorial Dynamics

Selzer handles this complication of the miscommunication by delaying its resolution, and, in so doing, highlights its significance. The character narrator, consistent with the mimetic representation of his relationship with Franciscus, does not report any further interactions with him after the scene with Imelda's mother. Instead, the progression jumps forward in time to the next morning, when the character narrator shows up to witness Imelda's family take her body away. With his own characteristic other-directedness, he gives Imelda's mother money "for flowers" and "a priest." She responds by praising Franciscus, calling him one of the angels and declaring that he "finished the work of God" and made her daughter beautiful (92–93). The character narrator is shocked, but when he looks for himself, he sees that Imelda's cleft lip has been repaired.

The character narrator's witnessing prompts the next two significant steps in the progression: his reflection on Franciscus's action and his imaginative reconstruction of the operation. Strikingly, his reflection moves from his perspective at the time of the telling to his perspective at the time of the action. He begins in the present tense and then explicitly calls out his shift to his perspective at the time of the action:

> There are events in a doctor's life that seem to mark the boundary between youth and age, seeing and perceiving. Like certain dreams, they illuminate a whole lifetime of past behavior. After such an event, a doctor is not the same as he was before. *It had seemed to me then* to have been the act of someone *demented, or at least insanely arrogant.*
>
> (93, emphasis mine)

The passage continues from his perspective at the time of the action, suggesting that "he had not done it for [Imelda's mother]" but because his arrogance meant that he could not accept the reality of what had happened. He ends his reflection this way: "People who do such things break free from society. They follow their own lonely path. They have a secret which they can never reveal. I must never let on that I knew" (94).

These serious judgments from the young medical student awed by Franciscus represent a remarkable change in his views. From his perspective, Franciscus goes rogue: unable to accept the accident as an accident, he attempts to erase it. And he doesn't seek consent from Imelda's mother but acts on his own. From this perspective, Franciscus's decision is the logical extension of the way he's always been. Selzer, however, invites his rhetorical readers to reach a different conclusion, namely, that the character narrator is unreliably interpreting and evaluating Franciscus.

Selzer guides his audience to recognize that the character narrator's reading of Franciscus as arrogant is not consistent with Franciscus's response to Imelda herself or with Franciscus's behavior in the scene with Imelda's mother, where he displays both humility and empathy. Even more revealing is that the character narrator's explicit interpretations and evaluations are not reflected in his imaginative reconstruction of the operation.

Since that scene is one the character narrator invents (I say a little more about this feature of the scene in Chapter 10 on Fictionality), he could have easily imagined it as one dominated by Franciscus's arrogance. But such arrogance is conspicuous by its absence. Instead, the character narrator's imagination produces a detailed vision of the care and respect Franciscus displays in that scene—for the morgue, for Imelda's body, and for his own work. The character narrator personifies the morgue, giving it a quiet agency consistent with its deep silence: "This room wears the expression as if it had waited all night for someone to come" (94). The character narrator also imagines Franciscus noticing a wooden crucifix on the wall, a perception that implies he's aware of being watched over by Imelda's God. As Franciscus sets to work, the character narrator imagines him as "stealthy, hunched, engaged" (94). Franciscus is attentive to every detail of the procedure, which culminates in "the most meticulous sutures of his life" (94–95). His exertions lead him to break a sweat. When he finishes, he does not cry out in triumph or otherwise congratulate himself. Instead, he simply collects his surgical instruments and leaves, allowing the morgue to return to its dark silence.

The gap between the character narrator's conscious reflections and his imaginative projection points to a gap between the character narrator's conventional understanding of medical ethics and his intuitive recognition of the change in Franciscus's character. Furthermore, the affective and ethical effects of the imagined scene are much more powerful than those in the passage of explicit reflection and negative judgment. Indeed, the effects of the imagined scene are consistent with the ones that arise from the scene between Franciscus and Imelda's mother. But the tension between the previously reliable character narrator's unreliable judgments and these affective and ethical responses adds to the power of this crucial segment of the progression.

4 Resolution via the Convergence of the Two Tracks of the Progression

The character narrator's concluding comment in his reflection "I must never let on that I knew" becomes newly relevant in the scene in which Selzer brings the two tracks of the progression together. Six weeks after the return from Honduras, the character narrator runs the slide projector for Franciscus as he lectures about the Honduras trip. All is routine until the character narrator sees that Franciscus has included a photograph of Imelda before surgery. The display of her face on the screen renders Franciscus unable to speak for a long time, and then he simply says "Imelda." He is clearly still feeling the effects of his encounter with her.

Since Franciscus has organized the lecture around the series of "before" and "after" photographs, the character narrator realizes that the next slide in the carousel must be of Imelda in the morgue. Rather than have Franciscus's operation on her dead body exposed, the character narrator removes that slide from the carousel. Franciscus gives the character narrator an ambiguous look—does it express gratitude or sorrow?—but he continues the lecture until the end.

With this convergence of the two tracks, Selzer guides his audience's interpretive and ethical judgments of both Franciscus and the character narrator. Why has Franciscus included the slides, given that they will not redound to his credit? The character narrator does not offer an explanation, but I suggest that Selzer invites his readers to fill in the gap along these lines:

Franciscus is still processing his encounter with Imelda and so he uncon- sciously opens up the opportunity to talk about that encounter. Be that as it may, his saying of her name and then being unable to continue reinforces her effect on him. She is, as the character narrator says, "the measure of his perfection and pain—the one lost, the other gained" (96). Again, both the action and the character narrator's representation of it invite rhetorical readers to recognize the significant change in his mimetic character, to empathize with his pain, and to ethically approve his acknowledgment of it.

As for the character narrator's choice, it is consistent with his character and with his intuitive understanding of Franciscus's own ethical action. He takes action to prevent Franciscus from the negative consequences that would follow from his revelation that he operated on a dead body. Selzer's rhetorical readers render a positive ethical judgment, but Selzer complicates the situation by introducing the ambiguity about Franciscus's judgment: did he look at the character narrator with gratitude or sorrow? In this way, the narratorial dynamics intersect with the plot dynamics: all the complications resulting from Imelda's death have now been resolved, but the ambiguity about Franciscus's judgment of the character narrator's action means that Selzer ends the plot dynamics on this note of ethical ambiguity. In this way, he invites his readers to dwell in the ethical complexities of that ambiguity.

5 Final Resolution and Farewell

The penultimate paragraphs complete the resolution and offer a farewell as Selzer has the character narrator return to the time of the telling. The character narrator summarizes the rest of Franciscus's life—he gradually withdraws from the surgical theater—and the corresponding changes in his character: he became "a quieter, softer man," who no longer went on field trips to Honduras or anywhere else (97). This summary emphasizes the radical change that Franciscus's encounter with Imelda and her mother has brought about. The encounters have robbed him of both his arrogance and his dispassion, two key lynchpins of his identity as a surgeon. Selzer guides his readers to regard these changes as positive: the lesser surgeon has become a better man.

The final paragraph is a farewell in the form of the character narrator's final reflections on his experiences in Honduras with Franciscus. Most notably, he reveals that he has changed his ethical judgment of Franciscus's decision to operate on Imelda.

> I would like to have told him what I now know, that his unrealistic act was one of goodness, one of those small persevering acts done, perhaps, to ward off madness. Like lighting the lamp, boiling water for tea, washing a shirt. But, of course, it's too late now.
>
> (97)

Rhetorical readers find it satisfying to see that the character narrator's articulate judgment now matches the intuition that guided his imaginative construction of the scene in the morgue. They find it satisfying, in short, to see the character narrator now offer reliable interpretations and evaluations. Furthermore, Selzer makes the evaluation clear and unequivocal (it was an act of "goodness") and the interpretation nuanced. The character narrator recognizes the limitations of Franciscus's operation—it is like boiling water for tea—and in so doing appropriately takes into account how small a gesture it was in the face of Imelda's death and her mother's grief. Finally, the farewell ends with an acknowledgment of something else that he is sorry for: he never did tell Franciscus what he thought, and he no longer can.

This ending, then, leads to a final reconfiguration of the story, one that brings Selzer, the character narrator, and Selzer's rhetorical readers into ethical alignment about Franciscus's actions in Honduras, and, ultimately, about his life. Affectively, the story evokes both a sense of satisfaction accompanying Franciscus's changed character and a sense of loss about his withdrawing from surgery. In that respect, the final reconfiguration includes a question: would it have been possible for Franciscus (or anyone) to have combined his brilliance as a surgeon with his late-arriving compassion for his patients?

Overstanding

This account of Selzer's story already includes multiple positive assessments, but I'll make explicit here what is implicit in the analysis to this point: Selzer's story works well on its own terms. But overstanding also involves asking questions about the adequacy of a narrative's terms. I turn then to illustrate how such an overstanding would work. I lay out a devil's advocate indictment of those terms, offer a public defender's response to that indictment, and then comment on the exchange from the position of an interested judge who does not have to rule in favor of the prosecution or the defense.

Indictment: The underlying ethics and politics of Selzer's construction of the progression are deficient because they rely on a series of ethically and politically objectionable assumptions. The descriptions of Honduras in general and Comayagua in particular are condescending and dismissive, expressing the attitude of a privileged first world author toward the third world. Both Franciscus and the character narrator share this attitude, as they implicitly regard themselves as white saviors of these Brown people. Furthermore, the most prominent assumption underlying the story is also the most objectionable: the white American male doctor's character and fate ultimately matter more than those of the Brown Honduran girl whose name Selzer uses to title his story and of her mother. Indeed, Selzer willingly sacrifices Imelda's life and her mother's grief for the sake of Franciscus's progress, or, to put it in other terms, he sacrifices their mimetic functions to their synthetic ones. Because Imelda is an Other, once she has fulfilled the function of giving Franciscus his moment of awe, she is dispensable. Because her mother is an Other, once she has fulfilled her function of providing a motivation for Selzer's operation in the morgue, she too can disappear from the narrative.

As if Selzer's constructive choices were not bad enough, consider these descriptions of Imelda by the character narrator that have Selzer's implicit endorsement:

> "A thin, dark Indian girl about fourteen years old. A figurine, orange, brown, terra cotta, and still attached to the unshaped clay from which she had been carved" (87).
> "As I watched, the mother handed down to her a gourd from which she drank, lapping like a dog" (87).
> "Set as it was in the center of the girl's face, the defect was utterly hideous—a nude rubbery insect that had fastened there" (88).
> "She was a beautiful bird, with a crushed beak" (88).

In other words, Imelda is ultimately subhuman, a clay figure or an animal. This representation is consistent with the deficient ethics underlying the construction of the whole progression.

Defense: The indictment of the condescension toward Honduras and its people is on point. The rest, however, is both overstated and too easy. These charges ignore both general principles of storytelling and some important context. The general principle is that narrative is inevitably selective, and part of that selection is typically about which character(s) to make the main focus and which ones to make subordinate. Yes, Selzer subordinates Imelda's and her mother's synthetic functions to their mimetic functions but he does the same with the character narrator.

As for the descriptions, they are metaphors Selzer uses not to dehumanize Imelda but to bring out distinctive features of her unmistakable humanity. In other words, saying that Selzer uses animal imagery stops too soon, and doesn't pay enough attention to its functions. After all, it's Franciscus's recognition of Imelda's humanity that makes all the difference: it generates his awe, and his sense of obligation both to Imelda and her mother. Finally, when Franciscus interacts with Imelda's mother, Selzer represents the interaction as a meeting of fellow sufferers, with Franciscus acknowledging her greater suffering. Thus, in all these ways, Selzer's ethics and politics are admirable rather than deficient.

Commentary: Let the debate continue. I expect that some readers will find the indictment more persuasive than the defense and others will find the reverse. And of course those on each side can bring in additional considerations.

I would add that engaging in overstanding does not inevitably lead to an all or nothing choice. It's possible to contend that the story is seriously marred by the bill of particulars in the indictment while also seeing value in the way the story works on its own terms. Furthermore, as noted in Chapter 2, when we move from understanding to overstanding, we also move from seeking consensus about how the teller guides their rhetorical readers to welcoming multiple perspectives on that consensus. In this way, rhetorical reading seeks to have the benefits that derive from reading in an authorial audience and from welcoming a diversity of well-considered responses to a narrative.

Opening Out

I hope that the detailed attention to understanding and overstanding "Imelda" not only provides a model for how to do rhetorical reading focused on character and progression but also clarifies and reinforces three important larger points about those resources: (a) progression subsumes plot; (b) character has three components—mimetic, thematic, and synthetic; and (c) the relation of those components in any one narrative is greatly influenced by the progression. Together these three points call attention to distinctive features of rhetorical theory that help it tap into both how narratives work and how readers respond to them.

More than that, I hope that caregivers and patients can recognize how the concepts of the mimetic and the thematic components of character are relevant to their interactions. Each recognizes the other as an individual (mimetic) and as a member of a larger group (thematic). Furthermore, sometimes the relation between the two components creates problems, especially when each looks past the individuality of the other in order to focus on their type. This problem often becomes acute when the caregiver thinks of the patient as a type of disease, e.g., "the stage 3 prostate cancer in exam room #1," and when the patient thinks of the caregiver as only their specialty, e.g., "the urologist in their office." When patients get reduced to their illnesses (or symptoms) and caregivers to their medical expertise, then the art of medicine drops out of their encounters, making the outcomes of their interactions less likely to be successful. On the other hand, when caregivers and patients pay attention to each other's individuality along with their group identities, they are likely not only to foster mutual respect but maximize the chances of successful outcomes.

With progression, the key point for caregiver-patient interactions is to attend to the way stories from either side move through time rather than to extract a single statement or other message. Narrative progressions in the clinic will typically not be as artful or complicated as the ones in our corpus of narratives, but even those told in the clinic that are apparently herky-jerky or even incoherent will signify something important. What is it that makes the narrative less than smooth or less than coherent? Being able to answer such questions on the basis of one's careful listening to progression can enhance the quality of a particular interaction and of the overall patient-caregiver relationship.

Springboarding Prompts

Again, the goal of springboarding is to build on overstanding and understanding, and, in so doing, to extend rhetorical readers' engagement with the story in ways that they find productive. These prompts, then, illustrate some possible routes to further engagement.

Rewrite Selzer's story from Imelda's perspective.

Rewrite the story from the perspective of Imelda's mother.

Tell a story about a turning point in your own life.

Tell a story about how you had to reassess and ultimately change your behavior.

Tell a story about how you observed someone you know undergo a significant change.

Tell a story about a time you broke the rules and the consequences that followed from your rule breaking.

Note

1 For a discussion of "Home Burial" as a lyric narrative, see Chapter 9 of my *Experiencing Fiction*. Part Two of the book is devoted to the concepts of portrait narrative and lyric narrative.

Works Cited

Aristotle. *Poetics*, translated by S.H. Butcher. New York: Macmillan, 1895.

Brooks, Peter. *Reading for the Plot: Design and Intention in Narrative*. New York: Knopf, 1984.

Browning, Robert. "My Last Duchess." In *The Norton Introduction to Literature: Shorter 12th Edition*, edited by Kelly J. Mays, 1103–1104. New York: W.W. Norton & Company, 2016.

Cisneros, Sandra. "Barbie-Q." In *Woman Hollering Creek and Other Stories*, 14–16. New York: Random House, 1991.

Forster, E.M. *Aspects of the Novel*. London: E. Arnold, 1949 [1927].

James, Henry. "The Art of Fiction." In *The Art of Criticism: Henry James on The Theory and Practice of Fiction*, edited by William Veeder and Susan M. Griffin, 165–196. Chicago, IL: University of Chicago Press, 1986.

Phelan, James. *Experiencing Fiction: Judgments, Progressions, and the Rhetorical Theory of Narrative*. Columbus, OH: Ohio State University Press, 2007.

Selzer, Richard. "Imelda." In *The Doctor Stories*, 83–97. New York: Picador, 1998.

Veeder, William and Susan M.Griffin, eds. *The Art of Criticism: Henry James on the Theory and Practice of Fiction*. Chicago, IL: University of Chicago Press, 1986.

4 Character and Progression II

Colm Tóibín's "One Minus One" as Portrait Narrative

As I mentioned in Chapter 3, not all rhetorical acts that we call narratives make change over time their central concern. Instead, some rhetorical acts subordinate their tellings of change over time to other concerns such as the revelation of character (portrait narrative), the exploration of an unchanging condition (lyric narrative), or the advancement of an argument (essay narrative). If this book were only about character and progression, I would devote individual chapters to each of these hybrid forms. But since I want to talk about other key resources of narrative, I will let this one on Tóibín's portrait narrative serve to make the larger point about the importance of recognizing that not all texts we call stories have the same forms. I will supplement this discussion in subsequent chapters, as I discuss Roger Angell's "This Old Man" as a lyric narrative in my discussion of its handling of time in Chapter 7, and touch on Ward's construction of an essay narrative in Chapter 11. I start by comparing "One Minus One" with "Imelda."

Tóibín's story is different from Selzer's in multiple ways: his character narrator is also the protagonist and, since he addresses a specific narratee within the storyworld who does not get to speak, the story has the form of a dramatic monologue.[1] Where Selzer uses the character narrator to offer a retrospective account of Franciscus and his actions, Tóibín represents the character narrator's address as it unfolds in the present tense. That address does include multiple representations of past events, especially ones connected with the death of the character narrator's mother six years ago, which in turn are connected to the way his mother treated him when he was eight years old. But the character narrator is in essentially the same position at the end of the monologue as he was at the beginning. Thus, there's a temporal movement of the telling and a corresponding temporal movement in rhetorical readers' understanding of the character narrator, but there is no accompanying change in him or his situation. Tóibín uses the telling of past events to contribute to his mimetic portrait of the character narrator. Like most other portrait narratives, "One Minus One" also thematizes many of the character's traits, and, indeed, sets up a feedback loop between the mimetic and thematic components of the character.

DOI: 10.4324/9781003018865-4

Since the character narrator addresses an ex-lover but Tóibín doesn't explicitly announce their gender and sexuality, it makes sense to ask about those traits. Knowing that the story is based in part on Tóibín's own life, and that Tóibín is a gay man who often writes about experiences of gay men, leads to the tentative hypothesis that the character narrator is also a gay man. More than that, Tóibín includes some textual evidence to support this hypothesis. The character narrator mentions that, after his mother's funeral, one of her friends, "who notices everything," refers to the ex-lover as the character narrator's "friend," "with a sweet, insinuating emphasis." It's telling that this woman does not say "girlfriend" and it's more likely that her emphasis would be used to refer to a same-sex relationship than a heterosexual one. At the same time, Tóibín's not calling attention to these character traits indicates his interest in subordinating them to others. The progression does not invite rhetorical readers to infer that the character narrator is the way he is primarily because of his gender and sexual identity. Instead, it invites them to infer that he is a gay man who is of special interest because of his particular history and current situation and the thematic points that can be drawn from them. A useful springboarding activity would be to see how the story would change if it were rewritten with the character narrator as female, heterosexual, or non-binary (and with the narratee's gender and sexuality changing accordingly).

As with my discussion of "Imelda," I find it helpful to summarize the big picture points before moving on to the more detailed analysis that follows.

- "One Minus One" has a global principle of movement across its present-tense telling governed by several global tensions (and gradual resolutions of them): who is this character narrator? Why does he only imagine making this phone call to his ex-lover? Why is the lover an ex? Why is his mother's funeral, which happened six years ago, the last "real thing that happened" (1) to him?
- It also has local principles of movement for the backstories, governed by standard narrative patterns of instability—complication—(partial) resolution.
- Furthermore, Tóibín invites the audience to recognize the causal connections among the three temporal periods of the story: what happened when the character narrator was eight, what happened when his mother died, and what is happening at the time of the telling.
- In recognizing and exploring these causal connections, rhetorical readers also come to see the detail in the portrait that Tóibín is painting: the character narrator is someone who has many appealing qualities but who ultimately suffers from an inability to form any lasting relation to others.
- Much of the affective power of the story arises from Tóibín's constructing a gap between what the character narrator recognizes about himself and what rhetorical readers recognize about him.
- The last paragraph offers especially remarkable strokes in the portrait.

- Tóibín's purposes in constructing this portrait narrative are to move his audience emotionally as they engage with the complex central character and with the multiple ethical and ideational issues related to him and his situation: issues about parent–child relationships, about the effects of childhood experiences on the formation of an adult's character, about the importance and risks of communicating openly and honestly, about home and longing for home, and more.

Let's take a closer look.

Tóibín's Introduction of the Global Tensions

The first tensions arise from Tóibín's adding a significant wrinkle to the standard situation in a dramatic monologue: the character narrator addresses not a present narratee but rather an absent one, someone who will never hear the monologue. The monologue is framed by a hypothetical—"If I were to call you, this is what I would say"—and so only Tóibín's audience gets to hear it. This wrinkle introduces the tension of unequal knowledge between Tóibín and his audience: why does the character narrator only imagine the phone call? What does this choice reveal about his character?

In addition, with this set up, Tóibín guides his audience to recognize that the character narrator effectively has two audiences, his ex-lover and himself. The character narrator uses the imagined address to the ex-lover in an effort to process for himself so much of what he is feeling as he talks: his ongoing grief, regret, woundedness, and desire for connection. In tracing that effort over the course of the whole story, Tóibín also guides his audience to see the character narrator more clearly than he is able to see himself, a vision that includes the realization that this effort has not been all that successful.

The next tensions are related: why imagine the call to the ex-lover rather than to someone else, and why is this person now an ex? Interestingly, Tóibín resolves the first part early on—in the story's fourth paragraph—but only gradually resolves the second part. In that fourth paragraph, the character narrator reveals that, at the time of his mother's death, he and his ex-lover had only recently ended their relationship (the ex-lover attends her funeral). Tóibín invites his readers to infer that the character narrator imagines calling the ex-lover because the character narrator cannot fully separate his relationship with his mother from his relationship with his ex and that, despite the passage of six years, he still desires some connection with that man. The consequences of the connections between the two relationships emerge gradually, with the most significant consequences arriving in the last paragraph, which I'll discuss later.

Tóibín introduces the next tension at the beginning of the fourth paragraph:

> If I called, I could go over everything that happened six years ago. Because that is what is on my mind tonight, as though no time had

elapsed, as though the strength of the moonlight had by some fierce magic chosen tonight to carry me back to the last real thing that happened to me.

(1)

This tension is one of unequal knowledge between Toíbín and the character narrator on the one hand, and Toíbín's audience on the other: what happened six years ago, why does the character narrator want to discuss it with this audience, and why does the character narrator regard it as the last real thing that happened to him? This tension lays the groundwork for the backstory that will resolve it, even as the narration frames that backstory as relevant to the character narrator's situation at the time of the telling ("that is what is on my mind tonight").

Exposition, Narratorial Dynamics, Readerly Dynamics

The initial exposition reveals the setting and the occasion for the monologue. The character narrator, an Irishman who now lives in New York City, is visiting an unnamed city in Texas. In that sense, he is twice removed from his homeland, and Toíbín will eventually make this sense of spatial distance correspond with the character narrator's feeling of emotional distance from his home.

Out walking at night, he sees the moon, which he equates with his mother who is "six years dead tonight" (1). That anniversary—and the strong association between moon and mother—prompt him to imagine calling his ex-lover in Ireland to rehearse the scenes surrounding his mother's death. Toíbín also uses this initial exposition to begin to guide his audience to draw inferences about the character narrator that he is not capable of. For example, Toíbín invites his audience to see a greater significance in the moon-as-metaphor than the character narrator does. In starting with the metaphor, Toíbín implicitly invites his audience to recognize that he is invoking the traditional association of the full moon with the maternal qualities of fertility and love and setting up that association to resonate throughout the story. The character narrator, who is not constructing the story but engaging in his imaginary phone call, shows no awareness of those associations.

The character narrator's initial address to the ex-lover is both considerate and intimate. He sets the scene, but also talks in ways that indicate that his audience doesn't have to be filled in about everything. He doesn't have to explain who his mother is, and he takes it for granted that he can wax metaphorical with this audience. In addition, rhetorical readers note the poetic quality of the character narrator's imagined address: the prose is full of alliteration, balanced cadences, and parallelisms ("so low and so full"; "six years dead" and "six hours away"; "asleep"). In this way Toíbín initiates his readers into the presence of a reflective and eloquent speaker, and in so doing, further draws them into an engagement with the first tension: just who is this speaker? At the same time, the speaker's eloquence, his consideration for the ex-lover, and his ongoing grief about his mother's death orient the audience to be sympathetic to the character narrator. Many of these elements of the initiation and their effects on the readerly dynamics deepen as Tóibín moves to resolve the tensions. But, as the monologue continues, the gap between what the character narrator sees about himself and what Tóibín invites his readers to see increases.

Backstories and Their Consequences

Key to the resolutions of the tensions are the two related backstories: what happened during his mother's final days six years ago and what happened during his childhood. When the character narrator was eight, his mother left him and his brother Cathal with their aunt and uncle for several months while their father was in the hospital. What's more, she never communicated with them during the whole period or said anything about why she didn't after it was over.[2] In addition to having the character narrator rehearse the events of these two periods of his past, Tóibín has the character narrator interrupt these accounts with present-tense comments about his relationship with his ex-lover. As noted earlier, the result is that Tóibín invites the audience to infer and contemplate the multiple connections among the three main times of action.

More specifically, Tóibín guides his audience to see that the character narrator's way of being in the world—that which makes him who he is, as son, as lover, and as ex-lover—was forged during those months when his mother all but abandoned him. He becomes someone who feels deeply about others but who is unable to express those feelings, because he has decided that doing so leaves him too vulnerable, too open to getting hurt. Furthermore, the character narrator only dimly perceives the causal connections that Tóibín's rhetorical readers do, and any time his perception starts to become clearer, he moves toward denial. These traits become especially clear when he moves from the backstory about his time at his aunt's to his present-tense reflections on that time.

> In the years that followed, our mother never explained her absence, and we never asked her if she had ever wondered how we were, or how we felt, during those months.
>
> This should be nothing, because it resembled nothing, just as one minus one resembles zero. It should be barely worth recounting to you as I walk the empty streets of this city in the desert so far from where I belong.
>
> (7)

The present-tense sentences are examples of unreliable interpreting and evaluating: the character narrator misreads the significance of his past and he moves away from acknowledging his mother's neglect. Tóibín implicitly highlights the significance of this unreliability by selecting his title from this expression of denial. At the same time, the character narrator's saying that one minus one "resembles" rather than "equals" zero indicates that he retains some awareness that the backstory is more than "nothing." At the level of readerly dynamics, this transition is especially poignant because Tóibín's audience simultaneously registers both the character narrator's ongoing suffering and his inability to fully admit its causes.

As the character narrator continues to reflect on the experience, he makes some reliable interpretations that he also links to his present situation:

> My brother and I learned not to trust anyone. We learned not to talk about things that mattered to us, and we stuck to this, as much as we could, with a sort of grim stubborn pride, for all of our lives, as though it were a skill. But you know that, don't you? I don't need to call you to tell you that.
>
> (7)

The move from the past to the present is as smooth as it is revealing: what I became then is who I still am now. Furthermore, the point that the ex-lover already knows him to be this way combines with several of the other present tense statements to resolve the tension about why their relationship ended. Especially telling are two other comments, one earlier in the progression and one that follows shortly after this transition from the backstory to the present tense.

The earlier comment comes right after the character narrator first refers to the end of their relationship:

> You know that you are the only person who shakes his head in exasperation when I insist on making jokes and small talk, when I refuse to be direct. No one else has ever minded this as you do. You are alone in wanting me always to say something that is true.
>
> (2)

Tóibín uses the juxtaposition of the report about the end of their relationship with this comment to suggest that the two are related. The character narrator's insistence on joking and his refusal to directly speak the truth mean that he keeps others, even the ex-lover, at a distance.

The second comment comes at the end of a passage about his feelings toward his mother:

> She loved, as I did, books and music and hot weather. As she grew older she had managed, with her friends and with us, a pure charm, a lightness of tone and touch. But I knew not to trust it, not to come close, and I never did. I managed, in turn, to exude my own lightness

and charm, but you know that, too. You don't need me to tell you that, either, do you?

(9)

Putting the passages together, rhetorical readers can see that the character narrator's relationship with his ex ended because the character narrator adopted his mother's way of being in the world as a response to her neglect. Like her, the character narrator uses lightness and charm to keep from talking about things that matter to him. Thus, Tóibín suggests, the character narrator has reproduced with his ex-lover the relationship his mother had with him, and the ex-lover has decided not to stay in a relationship in which he's always kept at a distance.

Six Years Ago

Just as Tóibín guides his readers to recognize how the backstory about the character narrator's childhood informs his relationship with the ex-lover, Tóibín also guides them to see how it informs the character narrator's experience of the events surrounding his mother's death. More than that, Tóibín emphasizes how emotionally wrenching the whole experience was for the character narrator. Tóibín frames the narration of the character narrator's mother's last days with his remarkable disclosure about his thoughts and feelings as he flies to Ireland:

> I began to cry. I was back then in the simple world … a world in which someone whose heartbeat had once been mine, and whose blood became my blood, and inside whose body I once lay curled, herself lay stricken in a hospital bed. The fear of losing her made me desperately sad.

(8)

Tóibín and the character narrator return to fundamentals: the initial union of mother and child, the child's consciousness of that union and the debt he owes to the mother; and then the child's natural feelings of deep, impending loss as he deals with the knowledge of her imminent death. I don't think I've ever come across a more eloquent expression of a child's consciousness as they contemplate the death of their mother. At the level of readerly dynamics, the passage evokes deep sadness even as it strengthens the alignment with the character narrator.

This moment renders what follows all the more distressing. The habits the character narrator developed in response to his abandonment and that have led to the end of his relationship with his lover keep him from directly expressing his feelings to his mother. These feelings include his regrets about not trying to get closer to her, especially when he knew that she was dying, and about not letting her know during her last days how he feels about her dying. But these feelings also include his assessment of her:

there was this double regret—the simple one that I had kept away, and the other one, much harder to fathom, that I had been given no choice, that she had never wanted me very much, and that she was not going to be able to rectify that in the few days that she had left in the world …. I touched her hand a few times in case she might open it and seek my hand, but she never did this. She did not respond to being touched.

(12)

Tóibín implicitly evokes cultural narratives about how parents and children reconcile when the death of one is imminent, only to roundly reject them. Instead of reconciliation via some breakthrough of honest communication, the character narrator experiences only this double regret. It's hard to say which is more heartbreaking, his realization of his own failings in his relationship with his mother or his conviction that "she had never wanted me very much." The last sentence of the passage encapsulates so much of what he has to regret: "She did not respond to being touched."

Resolution and Reconfiguration

At this point, then, Tóibín's portrait of the character narrator is both close to complete and informed by multiple emotions. The concluding sentences, about his feelings after returning to New York from the funeral, add the final strokes that not only complete the portrait but lead to some reconfiguration of it:

I understood, just as you might tell me now—if you picked up the phone and found me on the other end of the line, silent at first and then saying that I needed to talk to you—you might tell me that I had over all the years postponed too much. As I settled down to sleep in that new bed in the dark city, I saw that it was too late now, too late for everything. I would not be given a second chance. In the hours when I woke, I have to tell you that this struck me almost with relief.

(13)

Tóibín finishes with two big strokes. The first comes with the character narrator's reliable recognition—via his summary statement, processed through what he imagines his ex would say—that it is now too late for him to repair his relationship with his mother. This recognition is the culmination of his earlier remarks to his ex about who he is—the man who won't speak truth directly, who keeps everything light. The man with those traits evolves into the man who postpones too much and won't be given a second chance. Now he is also the man who possesses this knowledge about himself, knowledge that he has been living with for the last six years.

The second stroke is even more significant. The character narrator's statement that he woke up feeling almost relieved indicates that he has given up the possibility of changing. But here the occasion and the imagined audience for his monologue add more shades to the portrait and highlight the gap between his self-knowledge and the knowledge Tóibín gives his audience. The occasion indicates that his feeling of near-relief has not lasted, because here he is six years later reliving the past and re-experiencing his regrets. Furthermore, his choosing to process everything through his imagined address to his ex indicates both his desire to have a second chance with him and his inability to act on that desire. Rhetorical readers can imagine the character narrator conducting a similar imaginary conversation six years after this one. He is who he is—and who he is going to be.

With this final stroke, Tóibín makes the form of the dramatic monologue a significant part of its content: it contributes significant detail to the portrait, and it is detail that the character narrator perceives either dimly or not at all. His monologue shows that he is a man who both deeply desires the connection with his ex-lover and is utterly incapable of communicating that desire to him. Tóibín's readers recognize that to communicate that desire, the character narrator would have to be someone different, someone who could speak his truth directly—not just this one time but again and again as part of being in an ongoing relationship. In this way, Tóibín's completion of the portrait makes his readers' understanding of it even more poignant.

Opening Out

This chapter and the previous one point to the flexibility of narrative as a way of knowing and a way of doing. Authors can use it to do change over time, to do rich portraiture, to explore the many dimensions of a particular situation, and to add force to arguments or essayistic reflections. Furthermore, as authors do these things with character and progression, they are also engaging their audience's feelings, ethical values, ideas, and aesthetic sensibilities in ways that have the power to change their understandings of the world.

Caregivers and patients, then, should remain open to the flexibility and variety of storytelling in their interactions. Sometimes a patient's story will subordinate their experience with an illness to a self-portrait, just as sometimes a caregiver's instructions will be less about what to do and more about a self-portrait that provides an implicit rationale for those instructions. Caregivers who carefully listen to stories that don't follow the pattern of instability-complication-I'm-here-for-a-resolution can acquire valuable knowledge about their patients that can inform their plans for treatment. Patients who are able to draw out their caregivers enough to have them tell stories about themselves often succeed in increasing their caregivers' investment in their well-being.

Overstanding Prompt

Respond to the following claim: Tóibín's character narrator is so self-absorbed that he becomes insufferable—and so too does the story. Make the case for this position and then respond to it, agreeing or disagreeing, in whole or in part, and giving warrants for your response.

Springboarding Prompts

Retell the story from the perspective of the character narrator's mother.

Reflect on either how you responded or how you hope you will respond to the last days of a parent's life.

Tell a story about your own willingness or reluctance to risk being close to others by communicating honestly about your feelings.

Tell a story in which you use an imaginary phone call to talk to someone important in your life as a way to talk to yourself about something you care about.

Tell a story about your efforts to reconcile with a family member or close friend.

With the next two chapters, I shift my focus to a set of resources related to telling—agents of telling, first, and then key aspects of how they tell, though, not surprisingly, these resources cannot be completely separated from each other. But even as I shift focus, I will often find it useful—indeed, necessary—to continue to refer to character and progression.

Notes

1 Maura Spiegel and Danielle Spencer discuss "One Minus One" under the rubric of relationality in Chapter 1 of *The Principles and Practice of Narrative Medicine*. While they offer many sound points about the story, they do not offer the kind of detailed analysis I engage in here.
2 I note in passing that Tóibín brilliantly creates a character with the synthetic function of setting up the move from one backstory to the other. When the character narrator arrives at the airport to fly home to Ireland before his mother's death, he meets an airline employee, Frances Carey, who lived next door to his aunt and uncle when he stayed with them. That meeting provides the trigger for the transition from the story of the funeral to the story of his childhood. A thorough analysis of the progression would expand upon Frances's role in the story as well as analyze the roles of the character narrator's brother Cathal and his sister Suzie. But for reasons of length and clarity, I stay with the most important relationships, those between the character narrator and his mother, and between him and his ex-lover.

Works Cited

Charon, Rita, Sayantani DasGupta, Nellie Hermann, Craig Irvine, Eric R. Marcus, Edgar Rivera Colon, Danielle Spencer, and Maura Spiegel. *The Principles and Practice of Narrative Medicine*. New York: Oxford University Press, 2016.

Tóibín, Colm. "One Minus One." In *The Empty Family*, 1–13. New York: Scribner, 2010.

5 Somebody Telling I

Authors, Narrators, Characters, and Occasions

Narrative theorists have done impressive work on narrative discourse, and I'll get into some of its details later in this chapter and again in the next chapter on voice and perspective, and in the chapter on time. But for now, I want to highlight that the teller who has received the most attention from narrative theorists has been the narrator. Authors have gotten less attention due to other trends in literary theory, and characters due to trends within narrative theory itself.

Authors have been relatively neglected because both the New Critics of the mid-twentieth century and the post-structuralist theorists of the late-twentieth century have been hostile to them. The New Critics wanted to ground interpretations of literary texts primarily in the language of those texts. Consequently, they declared that interpreters who appealed to authors' intentions were guilty of "The Intentional Fallacy." (Terrible spoilsports, the New Critics also declared that interpreters who appealed to readerly response were guilty of "The Affective Fallacy.") Although no current critic or theorist claims to be a New Critic, the movement's anti-intentionalism has persisted. One reason for that persistence is that the post-structuralists went a step further by announcing "the death of the author." The post-structuralists wanted not only to keep the language of the text (and the semiotic codes that governed it) at the center of interpretation but also to liberate the reader. Rhetorical theory, as I hope is evident by now, rejects the implicit assumptions of these positions—namely, that paying attention to authors means neglecting the language of a text, and that readers can flourish only if authors die—and replaces them with the idea that authors, textual language, and readers can productively collaborate. This idea underlies rhetorical theory's conception of a feedback loop among authorial agency, textual phenomena, and readerly response as well as its Author—Resources—Audience model of narrative construction.

Furthermore, attending to authors also brings the occasion of telling into the foreground. Because this person opts to tell this story in this time and place to this audience, they fashion it in some ways rather than others. If this person were to tell the same story (that is, work with the same raw materials) on a different occasion, they would be likely to fashion it

DOI: 10.4324/9781003018865-5

differently. As would a different person working with the same raw materials on the original occasion.

Characters have gotten less attention as tellers as a result of the widely accepted distinction between story (the "what" of narrative, its events and existents) and discourse (the "how" of narrative, including techniques of all kinds). That distinction puts characters on the story side, and narrators on the discourse side, but a little reflection on the functions of dialogue leads us to recognize that characters also frequently function as tellers.

The Author—Resources—Audience model identifies authors not only as a constant in narrative communication but also as the ultimate somebodies of the telling, the agents responsible for the text being the way it is and not some other way. But authorial telling is typically mediated through the telling of narrators to narratees, the telling of characters to each other, or the synthesis of the two. Authors can also communicate through other means such as the use of paratexts (titles, prefaces, epigraphs, and so on) and through the arrangement—juxtapositions and sequencing—of chapters and other segments of their narratives. Let's take a closer look.

Authors and Their Reliable, Unreliable, and Deficient Narrators

From a rhetorical perspective, mainstream narrative theory's attention to the narrator (as distinct from the author) testifies to its importance as a resource, and, thus, to the value of recognizing the wide array of authorial uses of that resource.[1] Authors primarily use narrators to report, to interpret, and to evaluate. Thus, we can identify three axes of narrative communication, corresponding to each function: the axis of characters, events, time, and space (the location of reporting); the axis of reading or construing (interpreting); and the axis of ethics (evaluating). As we have seen with Selzer's and Tóibín's handling of their character narrators in "Imelda" and "One Minus One," authors can endorse their narrators' reporting, interpreting, and evaluating—or not—and can vary their endorsements over the course of a narrative. Further, they can endorse the reporting and not the interpreting or evaluating. And they can endorse the telling in one passage and fail to endorse it in another. And so on for all possible combinations among the functions. Endorsement signals reliable narration, and lack of endorsement unreliable narration. In addition, identifying the three axes of narration yields a taxonomy of three kinds of unreliability: misreporting, misinterpreting, and misevaluating. If we want to be even more fine-grained, we can identify three additional kinds for narration that is as good as far as it goes but stops short of being fully adequate: underreporting, underinterpreting, and underevaluating.

When authors use reliable narrators in nonfiction, some theorists say that the distinction between author and narrator no longer applies or, to put it another way, that author equals narrator. That position has the virtue of being clear and straightforward, but, from a rhetorical perspective, it is inadequate. Equating author and narrator obscures the author's exercise of their agency in relation to the narrator. It is the author who opts for using a reliable narrator and who makes decisions about how much to have the narrator report, and how to have the narrator express the interpreting and evaluating. It is the author who decides whether to narrate from their perspective at the time of the action (that is, the perspective of the experiencing-I) or their perspective at the time of the telling (that of the narrating-I).

Furthermore, equating author and narrator obscures the author's exercise of their agency in decisions that affect but are clearly not attributable to the narrator. For example, it is typically the author not the narrator who decides to switch from narration to dialogue and to divide the narrative into its distinct chapters or other segments. Rhetorical theory finds it better to use a scalar concept of *distance* as relevant to all author-narrator relations. We can then recognize that sometimes there is no distance along one or more axes of communication (reliable narration), and sometimes there is distance, and the degree of distance can vary (unreliable narration). In memoirs such as Tweedy's, we can also recognize that the author sometimes endorses the perspective of the experiencing-I and sometimes does not.

As the attention to interpreting and evaluating suggests, I find it helpful to distinguish judgments of reliability from judgments of objectivity. All narration is subjective, but only some is unreliable. Even apparently neutral reporting is subjective because language in use always has a tone. More than that, acknowledging that all narration is subjective goes hand-in-hand with the principle that storytelling always involves the teller's shaping of their raw material (characters, events, time, space, etc.) in some ways rather than others. Thus, when we separate reliability from objectivity, we understand judgments about reliability as judgments about the relation between two subjective perspectives, the author's and the narrator's. When those perspectives converge, we have reliable narration, and when they diverge, we have unreliable narration.

This way of thinking about author-narrator relations leads to a somewhat different understanding of the term "unreliable narrator" than one found in common parlance. There the term typically refers to a teller whose *reporting* can't be trusted for whatever reason. The teller may inadvertently misreport or deliberately lie about what has happened (or is happening). Caregivers often worry about whether their patients are unreliable narrators in this sense. From a rhetorical perspective, though, in these cases what stands out is that author and narrator are aligned: the teller is either honestly mistaken or dishonestly deceptive. Either way, the teller wants their audience to accept their narrative statements as reliable. Thus, such cases are in marked contrast to those such as we've seen in "Imelda" and "One Minus One," where the author establishes distance between themselves and the narrator and wants rhetorical readers to recognize unreliability. Consequently, I find it helpful to use a different term for these cases of mistakes and distortions: they are examples of deficient narration. I will elaborate on this distinction below.

How, then, do we determine whether a narrator is reliable or unreliable? This question is similar to: how do we determine whether someone we're in conversation with is speaking ironically? I'll identify some markers of unreliability soon, but I want to emphasize that, from a rhetorical perspective, there is no 100%-guaranteed-or-your-money-back method, because the communication of unreliability (or irony) works by someone *implying* to somebody else that the surface statement (or set of statements) is not to be taken at face value. The teller implicitly says to the audience, "I know that you know that I don't stand behind this statement."

This point leads to a recognition of just how remarkable character narration in general and unreliable character narration in particular is. The author uses the same text, addressed to at least two different audiences (the authorial audience and the narratee), to accomplish two different purposes (theirs and the narrator's). In this way, character narration is an art of indirection: the author communicates to their audience by way of the narrator's communicating to the narratee, and in unreliable narration, the author's communication diverges significantly from the narrator's, despite both relying on the same text.

Not surprisingly, even though there is no comprehensive list of textual strategies we can consult to determine (un)reliability, authors have over the years developed a repertoire of such strategies. Here are six commonly used ones:

1   Inconsistency. Narrators who say one thing about X on p. 2 and then say something else about X on p. 10 that doesn't square with what they've said on p. 2 are unreliable in at least one of those places. In "Imelda," the character narrator's judgment of Franciscus's arrogance does not square with his imagined account of Franciscus's conduct in the operation.

2   Departure from culturally accepted ways of reporting, interpreting, and evaluating. In Ring Lardner's "Haircut," Whitey the barber describes Jim Kendall's cruelty toward his wife and interprets and evaluates it as evidence of what an amusing person Jim is.

3   Telling about things that are either impossible or highly implausible within the rules governing the storyworld. In Ken Kesey's *One Flew over the Cuckoo's Nest*, Chief Bromden describes Nurse Ratched's ability to stop and speed up time.

4   Failure to connect the dots of the telling. Often a character narrator will report a pattern of some kind and either fail to recognize the significance of that pattern or misinterpret it. In "One Minus One," the character narrator is unreliable in this way. To take another example, in Kazuo Ishiguro's *The Remains of the Day*, Stevens the butler reports a pattern of his interactions with Miss Kenton the housekeeper that indicates that they are falling in love. But Stevens can't admit that to himself, to Miss Kenton, or to his narratee.

5   Signaling that a narrator's desire for something to be so overpowers their recognition that it cannot or will not be so. Joyce Carol Oates in "Hospice/Honeymoon," discussed below, uses this strategy to great effect.

6   Using a narrator's tics or what poker players call "tells" to signal unreliability. Two common tells are the use of particular phrases or sudden swerves from one kind of language to another.

Both unreliable and deficient narration can have a range of effects on author—narrator—audience relationships. By implicitly diverging from Whitey's interpretations and evaluations of Jim Kendall, Lardner establishes considerable distance between Whitey and rhetorical readers and that distance has estranging effects on the narrator-rhetorical reader relationship. Mark Twain's Huckleberry Finn also frequently misinterprets and misevaluates, but his unreliability has significantly different effects on his relationship with Twain's audience. Consider Huck's famous declaration, "All right, then, I'll go to hell," accompanying his decision to tear up the letter he wrote to Miss Watson so that she could find Jim and return him to his enslavement. Huck's declaration combines misinterpreting and misevaluating. But Twain has guided his audience to recognize that Huck's decision is the ethical high point of the narrative: Huck believes that he's condemning himself, while Twain's audience believes that he's saving both Jim and himself. In contrast to Lardner's creating estranging effects with Whitey's unreliability, Twain creates bonding effects with Huck's.

Dialogue

Authors use dialogue between and among characters for multiple, often overlapping, purposes. The three main ones are to reveal traits of the characters, to function as events that are part of the plot dynamics, and to report, interpret, and evaluate characters and events. When authors use dialogue for this third purpose, they are doing many of the same things they do with character narration. In a sense, character-character dialogue is character narration on steroids. In character narration we have one text, at least three tellers (author and each character), at least three audiences (each character and the authorial audience), and at least three purposes (those of the characters and those of the author).

Understanding character–character dialogue as involving an art of indirection leads to a helpful distinction between *conversational disclosure* (what characters communicate to each other in a scene of dialogue) and *authorial disclosure* (what authors communicate to their audiences through the conversational disclosures). This distinction enables us not only to identify the two tracks of communication in any dialogue but also to analyze the relationship between those tracks. This relationship can vary widely, from minimal distance (in cases where the author uses a character as a reliable spokesperson for his views) to maximal distance (in cases where the author communicates messages that run counter to the facts, interpretations, and ethical evaluations the characters deliver in the dialogue). Authors have multiple ways of signaling their distance: they can place clues in the conversation itself, and they can establish particular characters as unreliable reporters, interpreters, or evaluators so that whenever they speak, the audience's default assumption is that there's something off-kilter about their communication.

In addition, when we note that the author-audience relationship remains constant across all character-character conversations, we can also recognize another important communicative phenomenon, *authorial disclosure across conversations*, that is, what authors communicate to their audiences by means of the links between and among the scenes of dialogue. Authorial disclosures across conversations are the core features not only of plays but also of dialogue-heavy short stories or novels. Such disclosures become crucial to the dynamics of character-audience relationships (do characters know more than audiences or vice versa? And what follows ethically and affectively from these differences in knowledge?). Such disclosures across conversations depend upon the active inferencing of rhetorical readers, inviting them to connect the narrative dots and often to see more than the characters are able to.

At the same time, authorial disclosures across conversations are another site where the role of the unfolding responses of rhetorical readers influence an author's developing construction of a progression. Authors will rely on the inferences their audiences make on the basis of earlier scenes of dialogue in their construction of subsequent scenes. In other words, the underlying logic of the construction of a later scene resides in (a) the details of the character-character relationship in interaction with the specific occasion of the dialogue; (b) the author's assessment of what the audience has inferred from previous conversations; and (c) the author's assessment of what the audience needs to infer from this new scene.

I now turn to analyze the roles of authors, narrators, and characters-as-tellers in two different narratives, Damon Tweedy's nonfictional "People Like Us," the first chapter from his memoir *Black Man in a White Coat*, and Joyce Carol Oates's short story "Hospice/Honeymoon." In the next chapter, I'll add to these analyses by going into further detail on how Tweedy and Oates deploy perspective and voice.

Narration and Dialogue in Tweedy's "People Like Us"

In order to home in on how Tweedy uses narration and dialogue, separately and together, I will not do a full analysis of the progression of his chapter but instead focus on just a few key passages about his interactions with a white professor, Dr. Gale, during his first semester at Duke Medical School. But first a few words about the occasion of Tweedy's telling. Tweedy writes in 2015, at a time when he is a well-established psychiatrist, primarily about his time at Duke from 1996–2000. As a result, he positions himself as someone who has established himself as a doctor and wants both to give a thick description of his experiences and to thematize them in light of what he learned then and what he knows now. The occasion also enables him to reflect on what has and has not changed on the individual, the institutional, and the societal levels and to use those reflections as the basis for some proposals about how to bring about more beneficial changes.

Tweedy frames the account of his first interaction with Gale by noting that, after studying harder than he had ever done before, he had earned good grades on his first set of exams and was beginning to feel "comfortable, or at least what qualified as such for a first-year medical student" (12). The interaction occurs when he returns to the classroom after a short break in the professor's lecture:

> When I re-entered the lecture hall … Dr. Gale, our professor, headed in my direction. Ordinarily, he didn't socialize with students, so I expected him to walk past without acknowledgment. Instead, he stopped directly in front of me.
> "Are you here to fix the lights?" he asked.
> The sounds of the classroom seemed to vanish. So did my peripheral vision. Calm down, I told myself, maybe he was talking to someone else and only seemed to be looking at me. I glanced behind me. Nobody there. A few classmates were within hearing distance, but they seemed too engaged in conversation to notice us. Maybe with all the background noise I had misheard him.
> "Did … did you ask me about fixing the lights?" I said.
> "Yes," he replied, irritation creeping into his voice. "You can see how dim it is over on that side of the room," he said, gesturing with his index finger. "I called about this last week."
>
> (12)

In line with the previous discussion, we can identify four tellers here: Tweedy the author, Tweedy the narrator (the narrating-I), Tweedy the character (the experiencing-I), and Dr. Gale. Furthermore, Tweedy the author is the most dominant teller because he orchestrates the tellings of the narrator and the two characters.

Tweedy the author can choose to narrate from the perspective of the narrating-I (the narrator at the time of the telling) or from that of the experiencing-I (the character at the time of the action). In this passage Tweedy chooses the perspective of the experiencing-I. Compare a possible time-of-the-telling comment such as, "When I look back now, I still marvel at how powerfully that question affected my response" with the time-of-the action perception, "The sounds of the classroom seemed to vanish." By staying with this perception, Tweedy the author conveys the powerful effect it had on the experiencing-I's perceptions, thus heightening the drama of the scene.

Tweedy also magnifies the dialogue between the characters by refraining from including any explicit commentary from the narrating-I about it. Tweedy's decision not to include narratorial comments indicates his confidence that his rhetorical readers will be able to infer the authorial disclosures behind the conversational ones. Furthermore, Tweedy invites his readers to recognize the gap between Gale's understanding of the conversational disclosures and the experiencing-I's understanding of them. Tweedy discloses to his rhetorical readers that Gale's question has a subtext along the following lines: "Since you're Black, you can't be a student and so you must be a maintenance worker." Tweedy also invites his readers to recognize Gale's implicit assumption of power, his taking a first step to direct this Black person to do what he wants.

Similarly, by framing the experiencing-I's response only with his time-of-the-action doubt about whether he had heard Gale properly, Tweedy invites his audience to infer that the subtext of the character's question, "Did … did you ask me about fixing the lights?" is something like, "Why do you think I'm a maintenance worker rather than one of your students?" In that way, Tweedy also indicates that the experiencing-I heard the subtext of Gale's question. That communication becomes even more salient when Gale's next line of dialogue indicates that he has failed to hear the experiencing-I's subtext, as he continues operating with his initial assumptions about the Black person standing before him and the whole situation. Not surprisingly, Tweedy discloses that the Black first-semester medical student is a far better listener than Gale the white doctor.

I want to emphasize that the reason to identify the four tellers is so that we can become better listeners both to this passage and to other instances of somebody telling us that something happened. In this case, becoming better listeners helps us understand the relation between Tweedy's deployment of his three other tellers and his purposes in telling this anecdote. He uses the dialogue and his perspective at the time of the action in order to dramatize both Gale's racist assumptions and their effect on him then. And he wants to dramatize those things in order to demonstrate to his audience some of the obstacles facing him as he enters a largely white profession in a largely white institution, both of which are marked by Gale's casual racism. In this way, Tweedy effectively thematizes this startling incident.

Toward the end of the chapter, Tweedy tells about his second dialogue with Dr. Gale. Having responded to Gale's initial treatment of him by studying harder than ever, Tweedy receives the second highest grade on the final, and he then goes to ask Gale whether he has earned honors. Again, using the perspective of the experiencing-I, Tweedy notes that Gale recognizes him but offers no apology. After the experiencing-I shows Gale the high score on the exam, the passage continues this way:

> "Wow," he said, unable to conceal his astonishment. "I am very impressed that you scored this high. You've definitely earned Honors. You have nothing to worry about." …
>
> "Congratulations," Dr. Gale said, his excitement showing no signs of dimming. "This is really incredible. Would you be interested in doing research in my lab?"

In just a few weeks, I had gone from pariah to prize pupil. This unmitigated praise felt like another aspect of Stephen Carter's "best black" syndrome. The stereotype of black intellectual inferiority was so ingrained that for a black person to do as well, or better, than whites and Asians, they had to be "exceptionally bright"—earnest admiration and condescension wrapped in the same package.

(27)

In the first two paragraphs, Tweedy combines Gale's dialogue with the experiencing-I's perspective ("unable to conceal his astonishment"; "his excitement showing no signs of dimming") to further disclose aspects of Gale's communication that Gale is unaware of. In quoting Gale, Tweedy relies on the authorial disclosure across conversations to signal that Gale's praise is mixed with his persistent racism. Attending to Gale's dialogue in both interactions allows rhetorical readers to recognize that the subtext here is something like, "I'm astonished that a Black student could do so well in my course." Tweedy invites his rhetorical readers to supply the rejoinder, "And just why is that?" From this perspective, Tweedy's decision not to quote but to summarize the experiencing-I's side of the dialogue (he tells Gale he would think about the offer) is an effective strategy for highlighting Gale's self-incriminating voice.

In the third paragraph, Tweedy shifts from the perspective of the experiencing-I to that of the narrating-I. Here there is no interpretive and evaluative distance between author and narrator, as the narrating-I articulates the connection between Gale's praise and Stephen Carter's concept of the "best black." As he shifts perspectives, Tweedy moves from the strategy of gently guiding his audience's inferences about his experiences to explicitly thematizing them: this encounter with Dr. Gale is not just one between an individual white professor and an individual Black medical student but rather one that conforms to a larger pattern of structural racism. Both strategies—inviting rhetorical readers to fill in gaps in the telling and explicitly thematizing the events—contribute to Tweedy's purposes of conveying how his race affected his entrance into the medical profession.

Tweedy rounds off his narration of this meeting with Gale by telling his audience that he had no intention of working in his lab and writing, "I left Dr. Gale's office—the last time I ever saw him on Duke's vast campus—with a confused mixture of pride, relief, frustration, and bitterness. 'Are you here to fix the lights?' stirred then—and still today—each of those emotions" (27). Especially noteworthy here is Tweedy's use of the dashes in each of the two sentences. In the first, the dashes signal his switching from his perspective at the time of the action to his perspective at the time of the telling. That switch indicates not only that Tweedy followed through on his resolve about not working for Gale but also that the incident is well in the past. In the second, the dashes signal his blending of his two temporal perspectives. Most importantly, that blending allows him to powerfully communicate the ongoing effects of his two encounters with Gale. Furthermore, the very mixture of emotions shows that the story is not, as it might be in the hands of a more conventional teller, one of pure triumph or overcoming but rather one in which the outcome is permanently tainted by the racism that defines its beginning.

As this analysis indicates, my effort at understanding Tweedy's narrative bleeds into my overstanding: I find the telling skillful and effective, artistically marshaled in the service of Tweedy's important purposes. As always, however, other overstandings are possible, and I invite you to try out your own.

Bonding Unreliability in Oates's "Hospice/Honeymoon"

I turn now to another story by Joyce Carol Oates, "Hospice/Honeymoon," which will require us to shift from nonfiction to fiction and to consider unreliable narration. In contrast to the retrospective narration of "Widow's First Year," the tense of the narration here is either present or future. In addition, in "Hospice/Honeymoon," the protagonist's partner is still alive. In this respect, Oates's story provides a good example of the importance of occasion *within a storyworld*, as she traces the trajectory of an unnamed female protagonist's responses to the global instability of the story: the news that her husband must begin hospice care. At the same time, much of what I said in Chapter 1 about the occasion for Oates's writing "Widow's First Year" applies here. Having experienced the loss of her beloved partner, Oates turns to storytelling in order to offer to others insights into what it's like—or what it can be like—to undergo that experience.

As the title suggests, the space of hospice plays an important role in the story, but I'll defer a detailed discussion of how Oates handles space until Chapter 7. Here I'll just call attention to Oates's developing a contrast between the actual space of the hospital where her husband is being treated for cancer and the imagined space of their home converted into a hospice.

Oates shapes the progression to serve her purposes of revealing the powerful seductions of unrealistic optimism in the face of impending death. Oates begins with second-person narration: a narrator using the present tense to address a "you," who is also Oates's protagonist. Oates then shifts to the first-person future-tense narration of the protagonist in the second half of the story, as the second-person narrator becomes the narratee. Oates then returns to the second-person present tense narration in the final lines. Oates uses this sequence of tellings to give a rich texture to the complex affective and ethical dimensions of the seductions of unrealistic optimism and of the jolt that comes from recognizing their false promises. One effect of Oates's handling of the narration is to induce her rhetorical readers to succumb—or at least to recognize how easy it is to succumb—to those seductions.

Because I want to analyze unreliable narration, I will focus here on the protagonist's first-person narration, but I note at the outset that Oates establishes the second-person narrator as fully reliable and as having intimate knowledge of the protagonist's thoughts and feelings. In addition, the narrator treats the protagonist's struggle to accept the idea of hospice with sympathetic understanding. Indeed, the narrator and protagonist form a close-knit dyad, one in which each is well-attuned to the other.[2] This attunement in turn influences the readerly dynamics: rhetorical readers also sympathize with the protagonist's struggle and come to desire a happy resolution to it.

In the following passage, the narrator's attunement informs her second-person recounting of the protagonist's final steps to her acceptance of her husband's need for hospice (her husband has already accepted it). The narrator's account is knowing, kind, insightful (note the metaphor of metal filings), and respectful.

> Until a day, an hour—always there is a day, an hour—when you began to speak of hospice yourself.
> At first, you, too, are shy, faltering. Your throat feels lacerated as if by metal filings.
> Gradually, you learn to utter the two syllables clearly, bravely—*hos-pice.*
> Soon after that, you begin to say these distinct, deliberate words: "our hospice."
>
> ("Hospice/Honeymoon")[3]

The first-person section begins once the protagonist overcomes her initial denial that her husband needs hospice care, and in it she lays out her vision of what will happen next. That narration is also other-directed, but the main other is not the narrator but her husband. She does not address him directly, but everything she says is concerned with him and what she hopes to do for him. On the surface her narration appears to move toward a satisfactory resolution of the global instability, because the trajectory of the vision is from hope to optimistic promise. Here are the first and last lines of that vision:

> *It is my hope: I will make of our hospice a honeymoon.*
> *My vow is to make my husband as comfortable as humanly possible* ... .
> *Not merely* hospice *but our hospice* ...
> *For both of us, the "final days" will be a honeymoon. I vow.*

In between, the protagonist projects the details of her vision. Since the tense is future, the protagonist is not reporting but simultaneously interpreting (what it will be like) and evaluating (what values will govern her/their behavior). The vision is extremely appealing: she describes a vibrant space, dominated by their love for one another, especially hers for him. The vision includes the cooperation of nature ("*the atrium will be filled with morning light*"), a renewed physical connection ("*Of course, we will hold hands. His hands are still warm—strong*"), and her ability to supply him with things that give him pleasure: music, art books, food, visits from family and friends. As the narration progresses, the protagonist moves from simply accepting the need for hospice to warmly embracing it. Rhetorical readers, encouraged by the protagonist's move from denial to acceptance to embrace, commend these aspects of her vision.

Much of the protagonist's initial interpreting and evaluating is endorsed by Oates, because it is held in check by some reality principle: "*My vow is to make my husband as comfortable as humanly possible … . To fulfill whatever he wishes that is within the realm of possibility.*" She even corrects a rosy vision of him lying comfortably on the sofa, looking at the sky: "*Or, more likely, he can lie on a (rented) hospital bed, positioned in such a way that he can easily gaze out the window. And I can lie beside him, as I have done in the hospital.*"

But as the protagonist's narration progresses, it begins to lose touch with this reality principle: "*When he is at home, possibly his appetite will return. When I am the one to prepare his food, his appetite will return, I am sure.*" Oates guides her readers to recognize, however reluctantly, that the protagonist's leap from "possibly" to "I am sure" is unwarranted, one based far more in hope and desire than in probability. This clearly marked unreliable interpreting has two major effects: (a) it encourages a re-assessment of many of the previous optimistic details of the vision so that they are at least tinged with unreliable interpreting (e.g., "his lips, when kissed, never fail to kiss in return" now seems much more a statement of desire than a description of a reality); and (b) it sets up a clear frame of unreliability for the final lines of the first-person narration:

> *Not merely* hospice *but* our hospice. *Not sad but joyous, a honeymoon.*
> *We will be happy there, in our own home. Both of us.*
> *For both of us, the "final days" will be a honeymoon. I vow.*

Oates's abrupt return to the second-person narration removes any doubt:

> In fact, nothing remotely like this will happen. How could you have imagined it would!
> *Hospice*, yes. *Honeymoon*, no.

The second-person narrator plays the role of the good friend who tells unwelcome but necessary truths. "Time for a reality check"—and some gentle chiding. The narrator's reminder of the reality principle leads rhetorical readers to go further in their reconfiguration of the protagonist's narration as unreliable interpreting and to reflect on their own denial of the reality principle. Indeed, in that reconfiguration, Oates's readers recognize that the unreliability almost inevitably follows from the initial move to see honeymoon and hospice as equivalent experiences, or, to put it another way, to deny the difference between them. That difference resides in the interrelations between two primary features of each: well-being and time. A honeymoon typically has both in ample supply, while hospice does not. The final two sentences, which the typography suggests is a call–and–response between the two narrators, firmly re-establishes the difference between hospice and honeymoon.

But this unreliable interpreting has bonding rather than estranging effects because Oates endorses so much of the first-person narrator's evaluating of the situation: she will act out of love, she will be other-directed, she will seek what's best for him. This bonding in turn influences rhetorical readers' susceptibility to denial. Ultimately, because the misinterpreting arises from her love, Oates invites her readers to empathize with the protagonist even as they ultimately recognize her denial. This combination of bonding unreliability and interpretive and evaluative reconfiguration contributes substantially to the story's power.

Bonding Deficiency in Joan Didion's *Year of Magical Thinking*

In *The Year of Magical Thinking* Joan Didion tells the story of her life during the year after the fatal heart attack suffered by her husband, John Gregory Dunne, in December 2003. During that year, Didion had to deal not only with her grief about John but also with the stress of her daughter Quintana's life-threatening illness. Didion the author writes about her experiences with admirable frankness and insight, establishing her narrating-I as a reliable spokesperson and initially emphasizing the interpretive and occasionally ethical distance between the narrating-I and the experiencing-I, even as she insists on the continuity between them. Didion uses the narrating-I to expose the experiencing-I's "magical thinking," the various mechanisms she used to keep from accepting the irreversibility of John's death: if she doesn't discard his shoes, for example, then he will be able to return for them. This magical thinking is another version of the denial Oates explores in "Hospice/Honeymoon." As the narrative progresses, the distance between the narrating-I and the experiencing-I diminishes until, finally, they converge in their joint affirmation of John's lesson that "you had to go with the change" (232). Again, the occasion matters: the memoir appeared in October 2005, less than two years after John's death, which means that Didion's magical thinking is barely in the past even as she uses the writing to help come to terms with her grief.

Crucial to Didion's move toward going with the change is the experiencing-I's response to the autopsy report, a response that both the narrating-I and Didion endorse. This report, which did not arrive until "early December 2004" (199), is crucial because it allows the experiencing-I to accept that she was not responsible for John's heart attack, and with that acceptance she is able to extricate herself from much of her magical thinking. The problem, however, is that, for actual readers following one of the major threads of Didion's narrative, the endorsement of the experiencing-I's response to the report is, to put it kindly, difficult to accept.

By this point in the narrative, the narrating-I has reported that John had a history of heart trouble and of treatments for it, including an angioplasty in his left anterior descending artery in 1987. By this point, the narrating-I has also reported that the experiencing-I has been looking for evidence of something she or John could have done to prevent his heart attack. In fact, on the previous page the narrating-I has emphasized how strongly this search affects the psychic life of the experiencing-I: watching a television commercial that claims Bayer aspirin can reduce the risk of heart attacks, she "was seized ... by the possible folly of having overlooked low-dose aspirin" (206), even though she knows John is taking the blood-thinner Coumadin. Didion has the narrating-I conclude this section with these comments:

> As I recall this I realize how open we are to the persistent message that we can avert death.
>   And to its punitive correlative, the message that if death catches us we have only ourselves to blame.
>
> (206)

The troubling passage then begins:

> Only after I read the autopsy report did I begin to believe what I had been repeatedly told: nothing he or I had done or not done had either caused or could have prevented his death ... .
>   Greater than 95 percent stenosis of both the left main and the left anterior descending arteries.
>   Acute infarct in distribution of left anterior descending artery, the LAD.
>   That was the scenario. The LAD got fixed in 1987 and it stayed fixed until everybody forgot about it and then it got unfixed. *We call it the widowmaker, pal,* the cardiologist had said in 1987.
>
> (206–207, emphasis in original)

It is the clause "everybody forgot about it" that constitutes the deficient narration. The problem with the clause is not what it reports: the human mind has a remarkable ability to compartmentalize, and this forgetting can be read as another example of that ability. The problem is that, according to the unfolding logic of Didion's narrative, with its frequent and recent signals about the experiencing-I's quest to find something that could have been done to prevent John's heart attack, the admission that "everybody forgot about it" should not lead Didion to endorse the experiencing-I's conclusion that there was nothing she or John could have done. Joan and John—and his cardiologists—could have continued to monitor his LAD. Even if Didion wants to make the case that such monitoring would ultimately not have mattered, the way she has set up the passage both globally and locally requires her to make that case. To put this point another way, the deficiency arises from Didion missing the contradiction between the way she sets up the autopsy report and the way she treats the experiencing-I's response to it. Furthermore, Didion's choice to have the narrating-I quote the cardiologist's ominous words after John's angioplasty (*We call it the widowmaker, pal*) only underlines the deficient narration.

Let me come at the same point from another direction: why would I or any reader notice that this brief passage is deficient narration? As I read the memoir, the clause seemed to jump off the page because it ran so counter to the expectations and desires I had developed by attending to the shared quest of the narrating-I and the experiencing-I for something that could have made a difference. Attuned to expect and desire some resolution to the quest, I was stunned that Didion and I drew opposite conclusions from the evidence that provided the resolution. I submit that other readers committed to following the logic of Didion's narrative would reach the same conclusion.

Our understanding of the memoir's status as nonfiction supports this analysis, as becomes clear in a thought experiment of taking the narrative as fictional. In that case, readers who have intuited the larger system of intentionality would regard as unreliable interpreting and evaluating the passage's conclusion that "nothing he or I had done or not done" would have made a difference. The setup, with its focus on the search for what could have been done, and the conclusion, with its quotation of the cardiologist, would be sure signs that the author is signaling the narrator's misinterpretation of the report. Readers would be likely to conclude that Didion wants her audience to understand that the character narrator so deeply needs to end her search for something she could have done differently that she goes ahead and ends it even after she is presented with exactly what she has been looking for. Furthermore, this instance of misinterpreting would contribute to a larger design that depends on the development of distance between Didion and her narrating-I for the rest of the fiction. As part of this design, the resolution in which the narrating-I and experiencing-I come together in the conclusion that they need to "go with the change" would signify not an important stage in the working through of the experiencing-I's grief, but rather a short-circuit of that working through. This resolution would be an integral part of Didion's purpose of exploring the connections between mourning and self-delusion.

However, because *The Year of Magical Thinking* is nonfiction, this hypothesis about distance between Didion and the narrating-I is extremely difficult to sustain. In fiction, the author is clearly distinct from the narrating-I and the experiencing-I, while in nonfiction, there is continuity from one to the other. (The genre of autofiction, which includes such celebrated narratives as Karl Ove Knausgaard's *My Struggle*, separates itself from both fiction and memoir by disrupting the clarity of the relation between author and narrator: writers of autofiction deliberately leave their readers with questions about whether and when the "I" of the narrative is separate from or continuous with the author.) In Didion's case, the continuity between author and narrating-I gets expressed, first, in the alignment of the two figures from their common recognition of the magical thinking of the experiencing-I, and, second, in the gradual movement of the experiencing-I toward a union with their attitudes and understandings. It would be self-contradictory for Didion to intentionally undermine this movement at this juncture of the narrative. To put these points another way, the larger design of the narrative underwrites the experiencing-I's movement toward some partial acceptance of John's death. Consequently, it makes sense to regard Didion and the narrating-I as endorsing the conclusion that there was nothing that the experiencing-I could have done to have prevented John's heart attack. Thus, the off-kilter quality of the passage is unintended.

The discussion of how we might read the last part of the narrative if it were fiction is relevant here. But rather than Didion undermining the accuracy of the character narrator's perceptions, we have a situation in which the actual audience comes to doubt whether the experiencing-I's partial working through of her grief is as successful as the author represents it. The actual audience recognizes that the representation includes a remarkable shortcut: rather than face the big question that the autopsy raises—how could John and I have forgotten about the LAD?—the experiencing-I has evaded it, and the narrating-I and Didion endorse the evasion.

Nevertheless, many members of the actual audience—and I include myself among them—are likely to find that the deficient narration has bonding rather than estranging effects. It functions as very powerful evidence of the depth of Didion's grief and of her need to move beyond it. Didion's usual sure-footed self-presentation falters here. This faltering is eloquent testimony to the painful effects of the trauma of John's death and of the virtual necessity of denial. That testimony in turn makes the rest of Didion's construction of the narrative, with its various ways of naming, facing, and working through the experiencing-I's magical thinking, all the more impressive.

Opening Out

Practicing the kind of listening involved in tracking the relationships we have explored in this chapter is a great way for caregivers and patients to improve their listening skills. The relationships may include those between and among:

1   the somebodies who tell and the occasions of their telling
2   their perspectives at the time of the action and the time of the telling
3   conversational disclosures and authorial disclosures
4   reliable, unreliable, and deficient narration.

Furthermore, caregivers and patients can find a role model in the second-person narrator of "Hospice/Honeymoon" with her combination of sympathetic understanding and insistence on the reality principle. In addition, recognizing the possibility of bonding effects when tellers are unreliable or even deficient can expand our own capacity for empathy.

Overstanding Prompts

Respond to the following claim: Tweedy doesn't give enough allowance to Dr. Gale's own history and position and the ways they influence his behavior, and, thus, Tweedy constructs an unfairly one-sided account of their interactions. Make the case for this position and then respond to it, agreeing or disagreeing, in whole or in part, and giving warrants for your response.

Respond to the following claim: Oates writes an ethically deficient story because it manipulates its readers' emotions, and even punishes them for their positive affective responses to the first-person narrator's enthusiasm for her vision of hospice. Make the case for this position and then respond to it, agreeing or disagreeing, in whole or in part, and giving warrants for your response.

Springboarding Prompts

Rewrite the encounters between Tweedy and Dr. Gale from Gale's perspective.

Tell a story about a time when you were mistaken for someone else.

Tell a story about a time when you mistook someone for someone else.

Tell a story about a time when your desire for something to be a certain way distorted your perception of reality.

Tell a story about a time when you first confronted the mortality of someone close to you.

Notes

1 For a more detailed discussion of the theoretical matters I discuss in the first part of the chapter, see my *Living to Tell about It* and Chapters 5–6 and 9–13 of *Somebody Telling Somebody Else*.
2 Magdalena Rembowska-Płuciennik has proposed that the kind of attunement in Oates's story is the default model for second-person fictional narrative.
3 *The New Yorker* does not assign page numbers to its online stories, so I will not be able to give page numbers for my quotations.

Works Cited

Didion, Joan. *The Year of Magical Thinking*. New York: Knopf, 2005.
Oates, Joyce Carol. "Hospice/Honeymoon." *The New Yorker*, 30 July 2020. www.new yorker.com/books/flash-fiction/hospice-honeymoon. (Accessed 10 February 2020).

Phelan, James. *Living to Tell about It: A Rhetoric and Ethics of Character Narration.* Ithaca, NY: Cornell University Press, 2005.

Phelan, James. *Somebody Telling Somebody Else: A Rhetorical Poetics of Narrative.* Columbus, OH: Ohio State University Press, 2017.

Rembowska-Płuciennik, Magdalena. "Enactive, Interactive, Social—New Contexts for Reading Second-Person Narration." *Narrative* 30, 1 (2022): 67–84.

Tweedy, Damon. *Black Man in a White Coat: A Doctor's Reflections on Race and Medicine.* London: Picador, 2015.

6 Somebody Telling II

Perspective and Voice

In the analysis of Damon Tweedy's narration about his interactions with Dr. Gale, I noted that as author he shifted perspectives from the time of the telling to the time of the action, and I paid some attention to the way he juxtaposed Gale's voice with that of his former self. Similarly, in the analysis of Joyce Carol Oates's "Hospice/Honeymoon," I pointed to the shifting perspectives between the second-person narrator and the protagonist and commented briefly on their voices. In this chapter, I want to dig deeper into these two resources of narrative. After presenting some theoretical concepts, I shall return to Tweedy's and Oates's narratives to say more about how they deploy these resources. I will then offer a detailed analysis of how Edwidge Danticat makes them central in the construction of her remarkable short story dealing with both the dementia of one central character and the post-partum depression of another, "Sunrise/Sunset."

Back in the 1970s, the French narrative theorist Gérard Genette made the perceptive observation that the term widely used to refer to perspective, "point of view," actually conflated two distinct concepts: who speaks and who sees, later expanded to who perceives (see the whole discussion on pp. 185–194). This conflation was reflected in the way literary critics distinguished between perspectives simply on the basis of grammatical person: if the narrator says "I," they regarded the perspective as first-person, and if the narrator used "he/she/they," critics regarded it as third-person. (In the 1970s, critics had not yet paid much attention to second-person narration of the kind we saw in Oates's "Hospice/Honeymoon" or to first-person plural narration.) Genette's first move is to observe that any narrator, even one who typically uses "he/she/they" to refer to characters, can say "I," and thus the distinction according to grammatical person soon breaks down. For example, while Jane Austen is famous for her third-person narration, she occasionally switches to first-person, as in these lines from *Mansfield Park*: "Let other pens dwell on guilt and misery. I quit such odious subjects as soon as I can" (428). Given the inadequacy of the grammatical criterion, Genette contends that it is better to distinguish among narrators on the basis of whether they do or do not take part in the action they narrate. Genette uses the Greek terms *homodiegetic* for narrators who participate

DOI: 10.4324/9781003018865-6

in the action and *heterodiegetic* for narrators who do not participate, but I find it more user-friendly to refer to character narrators and non-character narrators.

Distinguishing between these two kinds of narrators is a good first step toward answering the question of who speaks. But things get tricky and sticky once Genette addresses "who perceives?" Genette proposes the term "focalization" to refer to an author's control of perspective and notes that authors have developed three main strategies:

1   They use narrators who are free to narrate from an all-knowing perspective. This strategy corresponds to "omniscient" narration, and Genette calls it "zero focalization."

2   Authors restrict the perspective to one or more characters. Genette calls this technique "internal focalization," and notes that it can be "variable" across a narrative. That is, some passages will focalize through one character, and others will focalize through another. As we'll see, Danticat uses this strategy in "Sunrise/Sunset."

3   Authors restrict the narrator's access to characters' interiority. The narrator only describes characters' appearance and behavior. Genette calls this technique "external focalization."

Most narrative theorists welcomed Genette's distinction between voice and focalization, but they were less happy with his taxonomy for a variety of reasons that I won't rehearse because doing so would take us too far into the weeds of narratological debates. It will be more productive to explain how rhetorical theory adapts Genette's proposals. Affirming the value of separating voice from focalization, I identify the five possible combinations of them.

1   Narrator's perspective and narrator's voice. Example: Tweedy's reflections from his perspective at the time of the telling.

2   Character's perspective and character's voice. Example: The first-person narration of Oates's "Widow's First Year" and the first-person section of her "Hospice/Honeymoon."

3   Narrator's voice and character's perspective. Example: In Frank O'Connor's "My Oedipus Complex," an adult narrator, using language appropriate to his maturity, narrates from the perspective of his childhood self.

4   Narrator's perspective and character's voice. Example: The first sentence of James Joyce's "The Dead" is "Lily the caretaker's daughter was literally run off her feet" (373). The perspective is the narrator's, but the use of "literally" interjects Lily's voice into the narration.

5   Blends of voice and perspective. The technique known as "free indirect discourse," in which a character's discourse is embedded within the narrator's, depends on such blends. The embedding is often signaled by use of third-person rather than first-person narration and by the use of

the past tense rather than the present. For example, Ernest Hemingway in "Hills Like White Elephants" reports the perceptions of one of the main characters this way: "They [the other people in the station] were all waiting reasonably for the train" (278). The adverb "reasonably" is in the character's voice, but the "were" embeds it within the narrator's telling. If Hemingway were to use direct discourse, he'd shift to the present tense: "They are all waiting reasonably for the train."

This focus on the possible combinations also posits two main kinds of focalization: external, referring to the narrator's perspective (#1 and #4); and internal, referring to a character's perspective (#2 and #3). Free indirect discourse (#5) can blend perspectives (and voices) or make quick shifts between them.

Lisa Zunshine has added an important dimension to narrative theory's understanding of perspective by attending to the ways that authors often embed one perspective within another (*Why We Read Fiction*, Part One). Consider the second sentence in this passage from Danticat's "Sunrise, Sunset":

> [Carole's] daughter, Jeanne, is still about sixty pounds overweight on Jude's christening day, seven months after his birth. Jeanne is so miserable about this—and who knows what else—that she spends most days in her bedroom, hiding.
>
> (n.p. in online version)

The dominant perspective here is Carole's. But, as Zunshine would say, Danticat embeds Jeanne's perspective within Carole's perspective. Zunshine would also point out that Carole's perspective involves her using her Theory of Mind skills, that is, the ability to attribute mental states to others on the basis of their observable behavior. Jeanne does not confess to Carole that she is miserable; instead, Carole observes Jeanne frequently staying in her room, and she concludes that Jeanne is miserable. For rhetorical readers the passage involves recognizing three levels of embedment: Danticat **knows** that Carole **believes** that Jeanne **feels miserable**. Danticat is also careful to have Carole stop short of identifying Jeanne's condition as post-partum depression. In that way, she creates a gap between what she communicates to her rhetorical readers about Jeanne and what Carole understands. I'll consider some other embedding of perspectives when I analyze the story later in this chapter.

Zunshine also brings in the cognitive concept of source-tracking or metarepresentation, noting that attending to the source of a perception influences readers' judgments about its likely accuracy (*Why We Read Fiction*, Part Two). Not all mind reading is accurate mind reading. Since Danticat is the author, readers know that she knows. Since Carole is a fallible character, readers know that her beliefs could be erroneous. Because Danticat shifts between Carole's and Jeanne's perspectives, she guides her readers to see that Carole's belief misses the mark: it is the "who knows what else" that depresses Jeanne, not her weight gain. Danticat also indicates that some of Jeanne's mind reading of Carole is off-target.

Rhetorical theory builds on Genette's concept of voice by expanding its scope. Rhetorical theory's question is, "who speaks with what combination of style, rhythm, tone, and values?" This formulation helps us recognize that the same speaker can use more than one voice and that different speakers can use similar voices. This formulation also begins to acknowledge that, applied to written language, voice is a metaphor. Furthermore, attending to voice means converting one kind of sense perception, seeing words-on-the-page, into another, hearing sounds-in-one's-ears. In that sense, skillful rhetorical reading of voice involves a kind of synesthesia. Attending to voice can also add to the pleasure of reading narrative by heightening our awareness of its rhythms (and its occasional movement toward music) as well as its implied values.

What do we hear when we listen for voice? Style—particular uses of diction and syntax that may or may not generate rhythm; tone—the attitude of the speaker toward the utterance; and values—the ideological and ethical dimensions of style and tone. This conception of voice builds on Mikhail Bakhtin's idea that language has multiple sociolects, and each sociolect is shot through with ideology. For example, the language of the medical school classroom is different from the language of the police station not only in its diction and syntax but also in its implicit privileging of its abstract, formal language (e.g., myocardial infarction) over the vernacular (jammer). And vice versa. Bakhtin argues that the novel is the most artistic genre because it consistently represents multiple sociolects in dialogue with each other, a condition that he called heteroglossia. (Notice how the term fits within the sociolect of the academy with its penchant for Greek terminology.)

Unpacking the workings of irony can give us further insight into how authors may use voice as a resource, especially how they can employ what Bakhtin calls double-voiced discourse. In irony, the voice in the literal statement gets undercut to one degree or another by another voice behind the whole utterance. Jane Austen's famous opening sentence in *Pride and Prejudice*, "It is a truth universally acknowledged that a single man in possession of good fortune must be in want of a wife," provides a nice example. Most rhetorical readers smile because they recognize that the sententious *style* of the opening with its formal declaration about "a truth universally acknowledged" builds to an anti-climactic and easily falsifiable naming of this truth. As a result, readers recognize that the narrator's *tone* is ironic: she is not endorsing the statement. Consequently, readers detect a clash of *values* between the voice behind the literal statement and the narrator's ironizing of that voice. The first voice belongs to those people—and Austen's reader is about to meet one, Mrs. Bennet—immersed in a marriage market that puts a premium on status and income. The second voice belongs to Austen's narrator who uses her style and tone to critique the values of the marriage market. And Austen implicitly endorses the narrator's voice.

Building on this analysis, we can redescribe unreliable narration as an instance of double-voicing: the narrator reports, interprets, and/or evaluates in one way, and the author guides their audience to hear their voice undercutting the narrator's.

Let's return to the passage from Gilman's "The Yellow Wallpaper" that we examined in Chapter 2:

> I wish I could get well faster.
>
> But I must not think about that. This paper looks to me as if it *knew* what a vicious influence it had!
>
> There is a recurrent spot where the pattern lolls like a broken neck and two bulbous eyes stare at you upside-down.
>
> I get positively angry with the impertinence of it and the everlastingness. Up and down and sideways they crawl, and those absurd, unblinking eyes are everywhere. There is one place where two breadths didn't match, and the eyes go all up and down the line, one a little higher than the other.
>
> (132)

Gilman double-voices the character narrator's telling. The narrator's style is direct, and her tone combines candor and urgency. She also values honesty and straight-dealing, as she indicates with her complaints about the devious patterns in the wallpaper, complaints based on her (mis)using Theory of Mind skills to attribute intentions to the wallpaper. Gilman's double-voicing undercuts not the character narrator's values but her interpretations. Attending to those misinterpretations also means becoming aware of Gilman's voice behind the character narrator's. A good part of the effectiveness of the passage—and of the story as a whole—arises from this particular kind of double-voicing: Gilman communicates the mismatch between the character narrator's admirable voice and its values, on the one hand, and her misinterpretations of her spatial environment on the other. This mismatch gives the character narrator's unreliable interpreting bonding effects. In addition, since Gilman increases the degree of the character narrator's misinterpretations as the story develops, she also increases the bonding effects of the unreliability. In this way, "The Yellow Wallpaper" demonstrates the peculiar paradox of bonding unreliability: the greater the distance between her interpretations and those of rhetorical readers, the more readers feel emotionally attached to her.

To consider a case of modulations within single-teller discourse, let's return to the passage from Angell's "This Old Man" that we considered in Chapter 2.

> Like many men and women my age, I get around with a couple of arterial stents that keep my heart chunking. I also sport a minute plastic

seashell that clamps shut a congenital hole in my heart, discovered in my early eighties. The surgeon at Mass General who fixed up this PFO (a patent foramen ovale—I love to say it) was a Mexican-born character actor in beads and clogs, and a fervent admirer of Derek Jeter. Counting this procedure and the stents, plus a passing balloon angioplasty and two or three false alarms, I've become sort of a table potato, unalarmed by the X-ray cameras swooping eerily about just above my naked body in a darkened and icy operating room; there's also a little TV screen up there that presents my heart as a pendant ragbag attached to tacky ribbons of veins and arteries. But never mind. Nowadays, I pop a pink beta-blocker and a white statin at breakfast, along with several lesser pills, and head off to my human-wreckage gym, and it's been a couple of years since the last showing.

(n.p. in online version)

Angell relies a great deal on his variations in voice to make his lyric narrative appealing. What those variations have in common at the level of style is a turn toward metaphor that defamiliarizes the experiences of aging: "keep my heart chunking"; "a plastic seashell that clamps" the congenital hole in his heart; "a table potato;" "cameras swooping"; a "human-wreckage gym." His tone combines concern with appreciation: "this is serious stuff but let me also register how amazing it is." Both the style and the tone convey the dominant underlying value of relish for life. That value comes through clearly in his parenthetical declaration "(patent ovale forma—I love to say it)" and in the otherwise gratuitous description of the surgeon at Mass General, but I suggest it's there in the lively energy of the whole passage. More generally, listening closely to Angell's voice allows rhetorical readers to realize that this old man is having a grand time writing about the stage of life typically dominated by the emotions of grief, loss, and impending mortality. Much of the appeal of Angell's piece arises from the way his voice pushes back on the conventional understanding of old age.

More on Perspective and Voice in Tweedy's "People Like Us" and Oates's "Hospice/Honeymoon"

Rather than re-analyze the passages I've discussed in Chapter 2, I invite you to do that in light of the previous discussion. Here I'll take up different passages, using the concepts from that chapter and this one.

With "People Like Us," we can look at Tweedy's handling of the rest of his first interaction with Dr. Gale. After Gale says, "I called about this last week," the scene continues.

Reflexively, I stroked my chin and looked down at my clothing to check if I seemed out of place. Clean-shaven, and dressed in a polo shirt and khaki slacks, I thought I'd done a decent job of looking the part of the preppy first-year medical student. Obviously I had failed.

"No," I said, stumbling to come up with a reply. "I don't have anything to do with that."

(12–13)

In the first paragraph, Tweedy uses internal focalization through the experiencing-I to capture his developing response. In addition to conveying his in-the-moment experience, this strategy again invites his rhetorical readers to infer Tweedy the author's larger points. The most salient of these are that for Gale (a) seeing race occludes his perceptions of class (he cannot see the "preppy" dimension of Tweedy's identity in the moment); and (b) Tweedy's race means that he cannot be a student. The voice in the first two sentences belongs to both the narrating-I and the experiencing-I, and it is restrained and patient, subordinated to the description of the experiencing-I's checking his appearance. With "Obviously I had failed" Tweedy continues with his restraint and patience but then ironically double-voices it. What's obvious is not that he had failed to look the part but that Gale had failed to see his look. By taking the blame on the surface, Tweedy makes his critique of Gale all the more devastating. Tweedy invites his rhetorical readers to recognize that underneath his literal statement about his failure is another one along these lines: "Obviously Gale couldn't see past my race and his assumptions about its meaning."

As Tweedy reports his character's speech, he sets up a subtle interplay between the dialogue and the internal focalization. That focalization again remains within the time of the action as it focuses on his response. In the moment, he stumbles to reply. And though the stumbling fits with his line of dialogue, "No, I don't have anything to do with that," that line subtly conveys additional meanings. First, it's a direct rejection of all the assumptions about race governing Gale's behavior in the scene. Second, it stops short of explaining his presence, inviting rhetorical readers to infer that the experiencing-I still wants Gale to see him as something other than a service worker. The rest of the passage confirms what rhetorical readers already know: Gale's racism renders him incapable of such vision.

He frowned. "Then what are you doing here in my class?"

My mouth went dry. Why had he intentionally singled me out in this way? Race was the first thought that entered my mind. I tried to summon an attitude of 1960s-era Black Power defiance, but what came out instead sounded like 1990s diffidence. "I'm a student … in your class."

"Oh …" he said.

Dr. Gale looked away, then walked off without another word.

(13)

With the first two sentences here, Tweedy again combines narration and dialogue to communicate more than the sum of each. He retains the perspective of the experiencing-I and embeds Gale's perspective within it (Tweedy knows that the experiencing-I believes that Gale thinks like a racist. And the experiencing-I is a reliable source.) In this way, Tweedy drives home his points about how Gale's racist assumptions govern his behavior. Gale frowns because this Black person whom he assumed was going to fix the lights has informed him that he's not here to do that job. Tweedy then switches to Gale's own voice, marked by its presuppositions of power, authority, and entitlement. "Here in my class" is tantamount to "here in my space" and the subtext of the question is along these lines: "I'm in charge here, and I demand that you justify your presence."

The experiencing-I, again a much better listener than Gale, hears that subtext and wants to respond with a challenge that would convey his own authority and power. Tweedy again uses the restriction to the experiencing-I's perspective to both capture his unfolding response and to add to the thematic component of the passage. Tweedy's reference to the difference between 1960s-era Black Power defiance and 1990s diffidence makes voice, and, more specifically, the history of Black protest speaking against dominant white culture, an issue in this exchange. With the move from the experiencing-I's perspective to his line of dialogue, Tweedy invites his rhetorical readers to see that the experiencing-I sells himself short. Although his voice is not defiant, it is direct, and direct in a way that reveals to Gale his own racism. Tweedy's "I'm a student … in your class" has the subtext "I'm here because I belong as much as the white students do."

Gale has no rejoinder but the weak "Oh …" Tweedy uses the ellipsis to signal that the authoritative, entitled voice can only trail off into silence, a point reinforced by the experiencing-I's noting that he walked off without a word. Gale's "looking away" is another detail of the experiencing-I's perception that Tweedy loads with additional meanings. Even when presented directly with what he has previously failed to even consider, Gale can't directly acknowledge it, let alone apologize.

With "Hospice/Honeymoon," I want to take a closer look at one passage of the second-person narration and one of the first-person narration, as well as at its closing lines. This passage of second-person narration marks a significant complication in the global instability:

> But, yes, you've heard. Must have heard. For the walls of the room reel giddily around you, blood rushes out of your head, leaving you faint, sinking to your knees like a terrified child, stammering, "What? What are you saying? That's ridiculous. Don't say such things! What on earth do you mean—'final days'?"
>
> Your voice rises wildly. You want to fling the cell phone from you.
>
> For you can't bear it. You don't think so. Not knowing, at this time, the vast Sahara that lies ahead with all that you cannot bear, that nonetheless will be borne, and by you.

This passage reveals much about the way Oates constructs the specific attunement between the second-person narrator and the protagonist. (I note in passing that this attunement goes beyond the narrator's using her Theory of Mind skills: a convention of this kind of second-person narration is that the narrator does not need to infer the protagonist's mental states on the basis of her behavior because the narrator actually knows them.) Oates makes the dominant voice the narrator's, a voice marked by its informal, familiar style, its tone of kindness and understanding, and its values of affection and respect. But Oates also makes room for the protagonist's voice, and, indeed, it's the narrator's framing of the protagonist's voice ("What? What are you saying?") that is the key to Oates's revelation of their attunement. The protagonist is responding to her husband's acknowledgment that he is facing his "final days." Listening to the voice without its framing, rhetorical readers register that its style is colloquial and familiar, that its tone is dismissive and commanding, and that its dominant value is life, or perhaps better, the denial of death. But listening to how Oates frames that voice within the narrator's sympathetic understanding, rhetorical readers register that the protagonist's voice implicitly recognizes the truth of her husband's acknowledgment. It's that implicit recognition of the truth that drives her resistance and denial.

More generally, Oates conveys the depth and texture of the attunement between the narrator and protagonist by giving the narrator the ability to shift from her own perspective and voice ("Your voice rises wildly") to internal focalization through the protagonist and free indirect discourse. With "For you can't bear it. You don't think so," Oates shows the narrator moving, after "For," to free indirect discourse: these sentences are the narrator's indirect renditions of the protagonist's "I can't bear it" and "I don't think so." Oates also demonstrates the narrator's sympathetic understanding by giving her the power of metaphor once she moves back to narrating from her own perspective and in her own voice. This metaphor blurs the line between time and space, as she compares the prospect of the protagonist's living through her husband's final days with a journey through a "vast Sahara" that the narrator will manage to survive. Oates invites her rhetorical readers to add to this prediction: the protagonist will survive because of her relation to the narrator.

Now let's consider a segment of the first-person narration.

> *Holding hands. Of course, we will hold hands. His hands are still warm—strong. His fingers, when squeezed, never fail to squeeze in return.*
> *As his lips, when kissed, never fail to kiss in return.*
> *I will sleep beside my husband holding him in my arms, not strong arms, in fact, rather weak arms, which nonetheless can be made to behave as if they were strong.*

The perspective and voice here belong solely to the protagonist. In that way, the protagonist's narration is significantly different from the narrator's because it lacks the narrator's certain knowledge, opting instead for attributing behavior and attitudes to her husband as part of her vision. Her voice is marked by her straightforward, informal style, her optimistic tone, and her valuing of love and life. Although Oates does not clearly and unequivocally mark the passage as unreliable interpreting—everything the protagonist reports about the husband's present condition ("his hands are still warm") and her own capacity ("weak arms") is reliable—Oates's earlier use of the narrator's metaphor of the Sahara desert (and other things) raises that possibility. To put this point another way, rhetorical readers can detect a tension in the passage arising from the relation between the optimism and values in the protagonist's voice and in the narrator's prediction about what it will be like to survive the final days. Furthermore, as we saw in the previous chapter, once Oates does clearly mark the protagonist's narration as unreliable interpreting, a return to the passage indicates that it shows her on the way to her more extreme denial that culminates in her equation of hospice and honeymoon.

Listening to these two passages in this way influences our listening to the final lines of the story:

> In fact, nothing remotely like this will happen. How could you have imagined it would!
>
> *Hospice*, yes. *Honeymoon*, no.

When Oates returns to the narrator's voice, she retains its knowledge and authority but, rather than highlighting its sympathetic understanding, she emphasizes its commitment to the reality principle. There's a faint echo of the protagonist's "What are you saying? That's ridiculous. Don't say such things!" but here there's no undercurrent of denial. And so the story ends with the dyadic partners' call-and-response, which, I suggest, can also be read as a chorus.

Perspective and Voice in Edwidge Danticat's "Sunrise/Sunset"

Edwidge Danticat's "Sunrise/Sunset" is a moving story, told primarily in the present tense, focusing on a mother, Carole, suffering from increasing dementia, and her daughter, Jeanne, suffering from post-partum depression after the birth of her son Jude. The title refers to a peek-a-boo game that Carole plays with Jude in which she puts a sheet over his playpen to signal sunset and then removes it to signal sunrise. But of course the title also functions for Danticat and her rhetorical readers as a metaphor for the difference between Jude's and Carole's stages of life. Throughout the story, Danticat demonstrates an imagination of both breadth and generosity as she skillfully draws on the resources of perspective and voice to represent the rich and different interior lives of Carole and of Jeanne. Indeed, by showing that the characters' disabilities—and their reflections on their conditions—are integral to their interiority, Danticat demystifies the dominant ableist idea of disability itself. In her treatment, disability is not some deplorable deficiency, something to be ashamed of or to be gloriously overcome, but rather something that naturally occurs in the course of one's life.

In addition to shifting between the perspectives of Carole and Jeanne (and embedding each woman's perspective in that of the other), Danticat includes a segment of backstory, focalized through the narrator, about Carole's childhood in Haiti. I will say more about this segment in Chapter 7 on Time, but here I note that (a) it further contextualizes Carole's perspective as a minority immigrant living in Miami; (b) it sheds light on why Carole's perspective is so different from that of her American born daughter; and (c) it extends the "sunrise/sunset" metaphor to Carole's life. Reading in the authorial audience requires rhetorical readers to take on these three different perspectives, that is, the narrator's, Carole's, and Jeanne's, to listen carefully to the voices of all three—and, above all, to attend to Danticat as the orchestrator of the play among the voices and perspectives.

Summarizing the plot dynamics provides a general context within which we can better analyze Danticat's deployment of perspective and voice. Danticat generates these dynamics from (a) the two tracks of instability—complication—partial resolution that follow naturally from each woman's condition; and (b) from the intersection of those two tracks: each one's condition adds to their mother-daughter conflict, which is also a product of their different life histories. Carole has lived a life of hardship and sacrifice, first during her life in Haiti and then again in Miami. Carole's sacrifice has enabled her and her loving husband Victor to give Jeanne a life of less hardship. The complications reach a climax on Jude's christening day, when Carole, misperceiving Jude as a doll, comes close to throwing him off the terrace of Jeanne's third-floor apartment. Danticat spares Jude, her other characters, and her readers from that disaster, but the event is also a signal that Carole's dementia is rapidly overtaking her. The story ends with her being taken from Jeanne's apartment by Emergency Medical Technicians.

As noted earlier, Danticat deploys variable focalization, starting first with Carole, then switching to Jeanne, then to the narrator for the backstory. I'll focus here on Danticat's handling of the internal focalizations of Carole and Jeanne because they provide the best illustrations of Danticat's perspective-taking, and because they are crucial to the story's overall effects. As for voice, Danticat fluctuates—sometimes within the space of a single paragraph or sentence—among the narrator's, one of the character's, and blends of the narrator with each of the characters'. Since my analysis here becomes fine-grained, let me frame it by highlighting the main points:

1   Danticat engages in imaginative but well-grounded perspective-taking in her representations of her two main characters and their particular disabilities. This perspective-taking includes the three levels of

embedment I noted earlier: Danticat knows that Carole believes that Jeanne thinks, and Danticat knows that Jeanne believes that Carole thinks. And the accuracy of Carole's and Jeanne's beliefs about the other fluctuates across the progression. By inviting her readers to share in that perspective-taking and source-tracking, Danticat also expands their capacity to understand the complexities of other minds.

2   Danticat uses the shifting internal focalization to track the further decline of Carole and point toward some improvement for Jeanne. The juxtaposition of these trajectories has significant multi-layered effects for the two characters and for Danticat's readers. In particular, even as Carole feels herself losing her cognitive grasp on reality, she recognizes Jeanne's improvement and achieves a complex resignation or even contentment. At the same time, Jeanne achieves a new recognition of her mother's situation, which prompts her to an expression of gratitude that would not have been possible at the beginning of the story. Carole's decline and Jeanne's improvement generate bittersweet emotions for rhetorical readers.

3   All these effects are further reinforced by Danticat's handling of voice.

Here's the story's first paragraph:

> It comes on again on her grandson's christening day. A lost moment, a blank spot, one that Carole does not know how to measure. She is there one second, then she is not. She knows exactly where she is, then she does not. Her older church friends tell similar stories about their surgeries, how they count backward from ten with an oxygen mask over their faces, then wake up before reaching one, only to find that hours, and sometimes even days, have gone by. She feels as though she were experiencing the same thing.

This entire paragraph is from Carole's perspective, and Danticat shapes her presentation of it in two especially significant ways. First, she starts in medias res with the instability governing Carole's track of the progression: the initial word "It" has no antecedent for Danticat's audience, but the use of "again" indicates that Carole knows what "it" is because she's experienced "it" before. By signaling that Carole is somewhere in the middle, Danticat immediately opens up the possibility that the story will trace her further decline. Second, Danticat gives Carole an awareness of her condition. Indeed, the passage as a whole shows Carole trying to process her experience of cognitive decline. And that presentation also opens up the possibility that one marker of Carole's decline will be her loss of that awareness. Danticat's use of the present tense reinforces this possibility. More than that, by giving Carole this awareness of her condition, Danticat adds another dimension to the global instability arising from it: Carole's own anxiety about its progress. Finally, by giving Carole both her self-awareness and the cognitive ability to draw the analogy with going under anesthesia, Danticat makes it easier for rhetorical readers to relate to Carole's situation and thus to take on her perspective, even as they recognize the peril of her disability.

The voice here fluctuates between the narrator's and Carole's, and it's not always easy to separate them. But I take the informality (in syntax and in phrasing) of "a lost moment," "a blank spot" as indicating Carole's voice and the more formal "one that Carole does not know how to measure" as indicating the narrator's. Similarly, the rhythmic effects of the parallel syntax in "She is there one second, then she is not. She knows exactly where she is, then she does not" indicates the narrator's voice. The style is clear and informal, the tone is serious and troubled, and the values privilege cognitive clarity over loss or confusion. By using the two voices and making it hard to separate them, Danticat suggests an alignment between the narrator and Carole, one that she guides rhetorical readers to share.

A second passage, in which Danticat shows Carole's thoughts about Jeanne, reveals how Danticat uses these resources to further complicate the readerly dynamics.

> Her daughter's psyche is so feeble that anything can rattle her. Doesn't she realize that the life she is living is an accident of fortune? Doesn't she know that she is an exception in this world, where it is normal to be unhappy, to be hungry, to work non-stop and earn next to nothing, and to suffer the whims of everything from tyrants to hurricanes and earthquakes?

Again, the whole passage represents Carole's perspective on what she takes to be Jeanne's perspective. (Danticat knows that Carole thinks that Jeanne doesn't know.) After the first sentence of free indirect discourse ("Her" rather than "My"), Danticat shifts, in the two rhetorical questions, to Carole's voice. One function of the passage is to complicate the conflict between Carole and Jeanne as it reveals Carole's negative judgments of Jeanne's alleged ignorance.

With the shift to Carole's voice, Danticat both guides her readers to go deeper into Carole's perspective and to recognize its limitations. Danticat orders the questions so that they move from a plausible expression of dissatisfaction about Jeanne's understanding of her place in the world to unfair complaints. The complaints are unfair not only because Carole's idea of "normality" equates her individual experience with the norm but also because she and her husband Victor have worked hard so that Jeanne's experiences will be different. In effect, Carole is holding Jeanne to a standard of the normal that Carole and Victor have tried to eliminate from Jeanne's life. As the passage progresses, then, it becomes more informative about Carole and her views than about Jeanne and hers.

In this way, Danticat guides her readers both to go deeper into Carole's perspective and to recognize its limitations. The progression to the second rhetorical question is especially telling, as Carole goes from an easy-to-accept, albeit pessimistic, view (it's normal to be unhappy) to the ideas that catastrophic events such as hurricanes and earthquakes are normal and that these events occur according to their own "whims." Danticat uses the diction and syntax to convey Carole's increasing sense of impatience and her attitude of complaint. The values of the voice are clear: my view of the world is superior to my daughter's. Carole is so invested in her own perspective that it overdetermines her interpretation of Jeanne's. Yet Danticat, through the earlier strong alignment with Carole and through the move from the narrator's voice to Carole's, guides her rhetorical readers much as authors do when they use bonding unreliability. Rhetorical readers recognize both the misinterpretations and misevaluations in Carole's perspective, but they also increase their sympathy for her.

Now consider this passage, narrated from Jeanne's perspective:

> Jeanne never wanted to be a housewife like her mother, but here she is now, stuck at home with her son. She doesn't leave the house much anymore, except for her son's doctor's appointments. Most of the time, she's afraid to leave her bed, afraid even to hold her son, for fear that she might drop him or hug him too tightly and smother him. Then the fatigue sets in, an exhaustion so forceful it doesn't even allow her to sleep. Motherhood is a kind of foggy bubble she can't step out of long enough to wrap her arms around her child.

In shifting the focalization, Danticat shows her skill at perspective-taking as she captures what it's like to be experiencing post-partum depression and invites her readers to take on that perspective. By juxtaposing Carole's and Jeanne's perspectives, Danticat guides rhetorical readers to compare and contrast them. Each woman demonstrates awareness of her condition and feels its force as something beyond their control. Each is deeply concerned about their potential negative effects on others: Carole, Danticat tells her audience, worries primarily about Victor, and here she indicates Jeanne's worry about Jude. Furthermore—and this point is especially striking—Carole and Jeanne have each observed the other's behavior and interpreted it, but each is unable to do the kind of perspective-taking that Danticat does—and that she guides her audience to do.

Carole has observed the multiple outward signs of Jeanne's depression, but she cannot recognize the depression itself, as her "doesn't she know" questions indicate. Juxtaposing those questions with this passage highlights the gap in Carole's understanding: "Then the fatigue sets in, an exhaustion so forceful it doesn't even allow her to sleep." For her part, Jeanne recognizes her mother's cognitive decline, but it is just another problem in her life. When Danticat first shifts to Jeanne's perspective, she writes this passage: "How do you become a good mother? Jeanne wants to ask someone, anyone. She wishes she'd been brave enough to ask her mother before her dementia, or whatever it is that she is suffering from, set in." The phrase "whatever it is" is more than just an expression of Jeanne's lack of knowledge. It also indicates that Jeanne's concern is less with Carole's suffering and more with her own missed opportunity. The sentence "She never wanted to be a housewife like her mother" indicates that Jeanne regards Carole more as a negative role model than as someone that she views sympathetically.

In short, Danticat opens up significant gaps—of understanding and of empathy—between Carole's and Jeanne's perspectives on each other, and even greater gaps between what she and her rhetorical readers perceive and what her characters see. Nevertheless, because Danticat guides her readers to participate in each character's perspective and because she gives sufficient backstory to render each one understandable, Danticat's exposure of these gaps creates bonding rather than estranging effects, especially on the affective layer of response. But these bonding effects make the gaps between the two characters more distressing for rhetorical readers.

As for voice, Danticat minimizes rather than maximizes the differences between Jeanne's and Carole's: Jeanne's move to metaphor in the phrase "a kind of foggy bubble" is similar to Carole's move to the figure of going under anesthesia. Given that Danticat's narrator summarizes things that happen more than once (the technical term is "iterative" as I'll discuss in Chapter 7 on Time), Danticat gives that voice more prominence in this passage. But here too Danticat frequently makes it difficult to separate the two voices (e.g., "Motherhood is") and thus emphasizes continuity between them, as she did with Carole and the narrator. To be sure, Danticat does not equate all three voices; the values expressed in Carole's rhetorical questions are not operating in Jeanne's voice, and sometimes the presence of the narrator's voice highlights the limits of the characters' perspectives. Nevertheless, by minimizing the differences in voice, Danticat does not erase or bridge the gaps in perspective, but adds to their poignant effects. These women have more in common than they are able to recognize.

Here's another passage from Jeanne's perspective, which Danticat locates right after Jeanne's conversation with her father about Carole in which Victor twice says that "we'll have to put her somewhere."

> Jeanne hasn't seen the pain in her father's face before, because she hasn't been looking for it. She hasn't been thinking about other people's pain at all. But now she can see the change in him. His hair is grayer and his voice drags. His eyes are red from lack of sleep, his face weathered with worry.

The conversation with Victor not only gives Jeanne an increased understanding of her mother but it also brings about another change in her perspective: rather than being overpowered by her post-partum depression, she now focuses on her father and his struggles. Danticat blends the voices of Jeanne and the narrator and underlines Jeanne's change through the progression of verb choices: "hasn't seen," "hasn't been looking," "can see." Indeed, while Danticat highlights the shift in Jeanne's perspective, she also emphasizes what Jeanne sees: Victor's pain. Furthermore, her perceptions are rooted in her own efforts at perspective-taking, as she uses her Theory of Mind skills to interpret Victor's internal states via her observation of salient aspects of his external appearance: hair, voice, eyes, face. This passage prepares the way for some larger change in Jeanne, even as Danticat brings into her exploration of Carole's condition its effect on others, despite Carole's efforts to minimize that effect.

The larger changes in Jeanne, appropriately enough, come in response to Carole and the dangerous situation in which she puts Jude. Danticat shows her actively analyzing the situation and orchestrating the rescue of Jude, actions that depend on her ability to accurately take on at least some of Carole's perspective. Danticat shows Jeanne modulating her voice in line with her efforts to see the situation from Carole's perspective. First, Jeanne appeals to Carole primarily as a daughter beseeching her mother. She addresses her primarily using Haitian Creole, repeatedly calling her "Manman" and saying "Souple" ("Easy") and "Tanpri" ("Please"). Then she switches to English, as she becomes the adult daughter claiming her baby: "Manman, please give me my baby." Note here that Jeanne is no longer "afraid to hold" Jude. Then, thinking that, if Carole doesn't recognize her, she should speak as an authoritative stranger, she says, "Let me have him, Carole." Carole finally responds to this sequence, as she says "Baby?" but in a voice that leads Jeanne to think that Carole is using it as "a term of endearment" directed at her more than a recognition that she is holding Jude. Jeanne seizes the moment, and soon her husband James is able to take Jude from Carole. Danticat does not go so far as to suggest that Jeanne's actions and her new perspective-taking signal the end of her post-partum depression, but they do suggest that she will be able to cope much better than she has been coping.

That suggestion is strengthened by Danticat including a remarkable passage in which Jeanne tries to read Carole's mind even more deeply than she did during the climactic scene. As Jeanne observes Carole being attended to by the Emergency Medical Team, she thinks:

> it seems as though she [Carole] were surrendering, letting go completely, giving in to whatever has been ailing her. She seems to know that she'll never be back here, at least not in the way she was before. She seems to know, too, that this moment, unlike a birth, is no new beginning.

Danticat signals Jeanne's focalization by repeating the phrase "seems to know," by using "here," and by using the vague expression "whatever had been ailing her." Given the progression to this point, Danticat endorses rather than undercuts Jeanne's perceptions, and, thus, Jeanne's ability to read Carole's mind is further evidence of Jeanne's progress. At the same time, what Jeanne perceives is difficult for her and Danticat's audience to take in: Carole is aware that she can't reverse her slide into dementia. The christening and its events, then, mark another turning point in Carole's life, one made more dramatic by the contrast between her and Jude: "this moment, unlike a birth, is no new beginning."

Danticat then switches to Carole's focalization for the remainder of the story, as she captures what may very well be Carole's last lucid moments:

> You are always saying hello to them while preparing them to say goodbye to you. You are always dreading the separations, while cheering them on, to get bigger, smarter, to crawl, babble, walk, speak, to have birthdays that you hope you'll live to see, that you pray they'll live to see. Jeanne will now know what it's like to live that way, to have a part of yourself walking around unattached to you, and to love that part so much that you sometimes feel as though you were losing your mind.

Danticat uses Carole's perspective and Carole's voice here, but again she communicates even more than Carole knows she's communicating. Danticat also takes advantage of the flexibility of the second-person pronoun, as it works simultaneously as synonymous with the impersonal "one" and as a substitute for "I." It also can be understood as an imagined direct address from Carole to Jeanne, one that shows Carole predicting what Jeanne's experiences will be. In addition, Danticat links "hello/goodbye" to the bittersweet meanings of "sunrise/sunset." And even as Carole focuses on the details of the hello/goodbye phenomenon of parenting, Danticat gives her a voice whose underlying value is love even before Carole explicitly names that love. Furthermore, in another use of the flexibility of the second-person, Carole's phrase "to love that part" of you combines her feeling for Jeanne and the feeling she predicts Jeanne will have. In this way, Danticat suggests that Carole has intuitively recognized Jeanne's improvement.

The story ends this way:

> "*Mèsi*, Manman," her daughter says. "Thank you."
> There is nothing to thank her for. She has only done her job, her duty as a parent. There is no longer any need for hellos or goodbyes, either. Soon there will be nothing left, no past to cling to, no future to hope for, only now.

Jeanne's words to Carole further signal her improvement. Aware that her mother may never fully understand her again, she expresses her gratitude in the voice of her mother's Haitian Creole and in her own American voice. That Carole doesn't reply signals her decline, even as her own thoughts recall the story's opening and her awareness of that decline. In light of her previous reflection on "hello/goodbye," that awareness includes her sense of reaching a stage where progress and loss are no longer relevant. But that awareness is accompanied by a sense of satisfaction at having completed something important: her job as a parent. The last sentence works as a marvelous blend of Carole's voice and that of the narrator, a combination of Carole's projection and the narrator's authoritative prediction. Sunset.

Opening Out

Let's step back and consider the layered lessons of voice and perspective in "People Like Us," "Hospice/Honeymoon," and "Sunrise/Sunset." The first lesson is about how Tweedy, Oates, and Danticat are themselves skillful ventriloquists and perspective takers. Their carefully shaped reconstructions or inventions (or combinations of the two) arise out of a commitment to the values of representing others' voices and taking their perspectives. The second lesson is about how they then guide their readers to listen to those voices and to share those perspectives, while also remaining attuned to their potential limitations. By following that guidance, caregivers and patients can enhance their knowing-how and their knowing-that. They can hone their listening skills and expand their capacity for empathy even as they learn more about the diversity of human experiences and the corresponding range of perspectives from which to view and evaluate them.

Overstanding Prompt

Respond to the following claim: Danticat's story is far too sentimental because it underestimates both post-partum depression and dementia. Her seemingly realistic story is ultimately a fantasy and as such it does more harm than good because it misrepresents what it's like to experience these disabilities. Make the case for this position and then respond to it, agreeing or disagreeing, in whole or in part, and giving warrants for your response.

Springboarding Prompts

Rewrite a segment of "Sunrise/Sunset" from the perspective of Victor or of James.

Tell a story about your relationship with one of your grandparents, parents, or, if you have them, children.

Tell a story about a memorable family gathering from the perspective of someone other than yourself.

Tell a story about your struggle to adapt to a new environment.

Tell a story about an incident in which you clearly misperceived what was happening.

Works Cited

Angell, Roger. "This Old Man." *The New Yorker*, 9 February 2014. www.new yorker.com/magazine/2014/02/17/old-man-3 (Accessed 13 December 2021.)

Austen, Jane. *Mansfield Park*. New York: Penguin, 2003 [1814].

Bakhtin, M.M. "Discourse in the Novel." In *The Dialogic Imagination*, edited by Michael Holquist, translated by Caryl Emerson and Michael Holquist, 259–422. Austin, TX: University of Texas Press, 1981.

Danticat, Edwidge. "Sunrise/Sunset." *The New Yorker*, 11 September 2017. www.new yorker.com/magazine/2017/09/18/sunrise-sunset (Accessed 10 February 2022.)

Genette, Gérard. *Narrative Discourse: An Essay in Method*, translated by Jane E. Lewin. Ithaca, NY: Cornell University Press, 1980.

Gilman, Charlotte Perkins. "The Yellow Wallpaper." In *The Norton Anthology of Literature by Women: The Traditions in English*, 3rd ed., edited by Sandra M. Gilbert and Susan Gubar, 1392–1402. New York: W.W. Norton & Company, 2007 [1892].

Hemingway, Ernest. "Hills Like White Elephants." In *The Short Stories of Ernest Hemingway*, 273–278. New York: Scribner, 1953.

Joyce, James. "The Dead." In *A Portrait of the Artist as a Young Man and Dubliners*, 373–412. New York: Barnes & Noble Books, 2004.

Oates, Joyce Carol. "Hospice/Honeymoon." *The New Yorker*, 30 July 2020. www.new yorker.com/books/flash-fiction/hospice-honeymoon (Accessed 10 February 2020.)

O'Connor, Frank. "*My Oedipus Complex*." In *The Best of Frank O'Connor*, 108–119. New York: Knopf, 2009.

Tweedy, Damon. *Black Man in a White Coat: A Doctor's Reflections on Race and Medicine*. London: Picador, 2015.

Zunshine, Lisa. *Why We Read Fiction: Theory of Mind and the Novel*. Columbus, OH: Ohio State University Press, 2006.

7   Time

Time and narrative are as intertwined as the dancer and the dance. In addressing "The Power of Narrative" in Chapter 1, I began by stating that "We use narrative to make sense of our experiences in and of the world, especially our experiences of time and change." The philosopher Paul Ricœur has famously declared that "time becomes human ... to the extent that it is organized after the manner of a narrative; narrative, in turn, is meaningful to the extent that it portrays the features of temporal experience."[1] Not surprisingly, then, commentary on time has crept into every chapter of this book, and, indeed, it is essential for talking about occasion, progression, and perspective. When something is told has consequences for how it is told and how it is received. The importance of progression is rooted in the idea that narrative is a telling about time that unfolds over time. Perspective highlights the significant differences between time of the action and time of the telling. In terms of the progression of this book, it is, well, high time to give this resource its own chapter. I will focus here on how time itself gets represented in narrative, though inevitably the discussion will touch on issues of occasion, perspective, and progression. I will begin with some general points that I illustrate with reference to Tobias Wolff's "Close Calls" as well as to several narratives I've previously discussed. I will then do a somewhat longer discussion of a passage from "Sunrise/Sunset," and then spend more time with Roger Angell's handling of time in his nonfictional lyric narrative "This Old Man."

Time is central to narrative because it's central to the ways humans think about their lives. Different cultures have different conceptions of time, but no culture that I'm aware of is without any conception of it, if only because all cultures need a way to think about birth and death. In the West, we divide time into past, present, and future, a division reinforced by clock time. Clock time moves in only one direction—forward into the future—and it does so at a constant pace. When we say that it is midnight, we know that 11:59:59 is the past and 12:00:01 is the future. And because time only moves forward, we know that in a minute midnight will be the past and 12:01:00 will be the present.

DOI: 10.4324/9781003018865-7

When we give our age, we foreground the present but also implicitly include the past and the future. When we write today's date, we do the same thing on a larger scale.

Given that clock time is so deeply ingrained in our experience of the world, you may be surprised to learn that few narratives, and almost no narratives of any great length, are bound by the strictures of clock time. Homer's *Iliad*, often cited as the first major narrative in the Western tradition, famously begins in medias res. Julius Caesar's "veni, vidi, vici" ("I came, I saw, I conquered"), which we glanced at in Chapter 1, is the exception that proves the rule. When Caesar tells a longer story in his *Commentaries on the Gallic Wars*, he departs from straight chronological telling.

The discrepancy between clock time and time in narrative results from the way humans use narrative as way of knowing and a way of doing. Humans experience time subjectively, which is to say that our experience of time often does not match the passing of time on the clock. Sometimes a minute will feel like an hour, and sometimes a day will feel like a minute. In order to come to terms with our experiences and in order to influence others, narrative needs to be flexible in its handling of time. Sometimes (!) we need to skip over experiences or give short summaries of experiences that stretched out over long intervals of time in order to get at what we regard as the most significant parts of our experiences. On other occasions we need to dwell for a long time in our telling on experiences that lasted only a short time. In addition, to understand where we are now, we typically need to understand the past and to project a future. In other words, in telling about the present, we often need to look back and to look ahead. To take a simple example, consider this declaration: "I am a better listener now than I was when I started reading this book, but I'll be twice as good when I finish it next week." Rooted in the present ("I am"), the speaker clearly and efficiently assesses their progress by reference to the recent past ("when I started") and the near future ("next week").

Not surprisingly, narrative theory has done valuable work on time in narrative. Once again Gérard Genette has done foundational work, so I'll focus on his proposals about time in narrative and then discuss how I integrate them into a conception of narrative as rhetoric. Genette highlights three major aspects of temporality: order, duration, and frequency. He conceptualizes each one as involving a relation between "story time," that is, the underlying chronology of events in a narrative, and "discourse time," that is, the representation of those events in the narrative text. Here's a closer look.

With order, Genette posits that the default setting is to match the sequence of events in the told with their sequence in the telling. In "Close Calls," Wolff tells about three times when he almost lost his life, and his telling follows the order of their occurrence during his tour of duty in Vietnam. But Genette is more interested in identifying and discussing the two main kinds of mismatches between the order of the told and that of the telling: analepsis and prolepsis. Genette defines analepsis this way: "any evocation after the fact of an event that took place earlier than the point in the story where we are at any given moment" (40). This formulation, "any evocation after the fact," means that the more common term "flashback" is not an exact synonym for "analepsis" but rather identifies one frequently used kind. Flashback typically refers to the narration of an event or a series of events. Thus, in a statement such as "I love you more today than yesterday," most people would say that we have an analepsis (everything after "than") but not a flashback. The same logic applies to prolepsis and flashforward.

Crucial to Genette's account is the additional concept of "first narrative" (48), which for the sake of clarity I will amend to "primary narrative": the events whose progress constitutes the narrative now, whether narrated in the present, past, or even future tense. Thus, in "One Minus One," the primary narrative is the unfolding imaginary phone call, and the character narrator's accounts of what happened when he was eight years old and what happened when he visited his mother in her last days are analepses (and these analepses are flashbacks). In "Close Calls," the primary narrative is that chronological account of Wolff's brushes with death, but Wolff embeds an analepsis in his telling about the third close call. In this case, an arbitrary choice by a commanding officer leads to another soldier, Keith Young, dying instead of Wolff. After narrating the incident itself, Wolff flashes back to a scene in which he accompanied the enthusiastic Keith to a tailor who was to give them both an allegedly great deal on suits. Wolff returns to the primary narrative by saying that when he learned of Keith's death, he immediately thought of the suits. This move from the primary narrative to the past and then back to narrative now emphasizes how deeply the close call affected Wolff. I'll have more to say about this third brush with death in Chapter 10 on Fictionality.

If we want to get even more fine-grained, we can also differentiate the two analepses in "One Minus One" according to what Genette calls their *reach*, i.e., the temporal distance between the narrative now and the analepsis, and their *extent*, i.e., the length of time narrated in it. Thus, the analepsis to childhood has both a greater reach (it occurred many years before the mother's death) and a greater extent (months rather than days). In addition, both analepses are to events that are completed before the primary narrative and thus are what Genette calls *external* analepses. Finally, we can note that the analepsis about childhood is itself embedded within the analepsis about his mother's death, and that the character narrator frequently moves from present to past and back again. In "Close Calls," the reach of the analepsis is only a few months and the extent only a couple of days. But, as we'll see in Chapter 10, Wolff connects it not only with the primary narrative about his close calls but with the time of the telling. The overall effect of Tóibín's and Wolff's handling of the analepses is to emphasize the layering of past on the present, the way in which each one offers his own version of William Faulkner's famous claim that "The past is not dead. It is not even past." Needless to say, not all authors handle analepses in this way.

Since narrative is often told in the past tense, we should distinguish analepsis from retrospection. Retrospection, signaled by the past tense, is the default stance of narrative, because, as Dorrit Cohn puts it, "we live now and tell later" (96). In other words, we make sense of experience (our own and others') by telling stories about it after we've had it. Thus, analepsis typically occurs within the retrospection of narration, as it does in Tweedy's "People Like Us." Tweedy's first sentence begins the primary narrative in the past tense: "It was a late summer morning, a month into my first year as a Duke medical student." But then he employs analepsis to provide the larger context, telling about his family background, about his initial struggles to feel like he belonged at Duke, and about his recently feeling better about his situation. Then he returns to the primary narrative and narrates his encounter with Dr. Gale. In that sense, his analepsis is a retrospection within a retrospection. In the same way, Wolff's analepsis about his suit-buying excursion with Keith is a retrospection within a retrospection.

The first step toward integrating Genette's ideas about analepsis into rhetorical theory is to notice that *what is retrospective for the teller is part of an unfolding present for the reader.* As the teller (in the default mode of narrative) looks back on what has happened, the reader looks forward to what will happen next. In other words, while analepsis from the perspective of the teller is a retrospection within a retrospection, a circumscribed looking back within the global looking back of the primary narrative, analepsis from the perspective of the reader is both a looking back from the unfolding present of the primary narrative and part of the relentlessly forward movement of the act of reading. Foregrounding this paradox again highlights the importance of *narrative progression* with its attention to the synthesis of textual and readerly dynamics for a rhetorical conception of narrative. Reading for progression means noticing both the analeptic move in the textual dynamics and the consequences of that move for the audience's developing multi-layered response. In the case of Tweedy's "People Like Us," the analepsis deepens rhetorical readers' sympathy for and ethically positive judgments of Tweedy the character and sharpens their negative ethical judgments of Dr. Gale.

Prolepsis initially appears to be the mirror image of analepsis: the evocation *before* the fact of an event that will take place (or is predicted to take place) *later than* the point in the story we have currently reached. From the perspective of the teller and of textual dynamics, this description is apt. If analepsis is typically a retrospection within a retrospection, prolepsis is typically an anticipation within that retrospection.

When we shift to the perspective of the reader and the concerns of readerly dynamics, however, the metaphor of prolepsis as the mirror image of analepsis becomes only partially apt. The mirror metaphor implies that just as analepsis depends on the principle that an understanding of the past is necessary to an understanding of the (unfolding) present, so too does prolepsis depend on the principle that an understanding of the future is necessary to an understanding of that (unfolding) present. To be sure, that principle often applies and in cases such as the character narrator's projecting a future in "Hospice/Honeymoon" it is the most important one. In Oates's story, the character narrator's evocation of future events ultimately reveals way more about her current situation than it does about what will happen. But sometimes prolepsis, when delivered with the authority of a reliable narrator, does much more than shed light on the unfolding present precisely because its revelations are about the future. In this respect, the prolepsis works by a principle of bonus revelation about that future: "out of all the possible futures that you readers might project from this moment in the unfolding narrative, here is the one that occurred."

In the narratives considered so far, the best example is from the ending of Danticat's "Sunrise/Sunset," when Carole thinks that "Jeanne will now know what it's like to live that way, to have a part of yourself walking around unattached to you, and to love that part so much that you sometimes feel as though you were losing your mind." To be sure, since this prolepsis is located in Carole's perspective rather than the narrator's, it is a provisional one that also functions to shed light on Carole's present situation. But given the other signs of Jeanne's change, Danticat invites her audience to take it as a bonus revelation about Jeanne's future. The effect of the proleptic bonus is to shift the emphasis of readerly concerns from "what" will happen to Jeanne and Jude to "how and with what other consequences?"

With frequency, Genette homes in on the relation between the number of times something happens in the story and the number of times it gets narrated in the discourse (113–160). Authors have worked with all four possible relations: something that happens once in story time gets narrated once; something that happens multiple times gets narrated multiple times; something that happens multiple times gets narrated once; something that happens once gets narrated multiple times. (Genette is aware of the fifth possibility, something happening once or multiple times but not getting narrated at all, but, as I note later, he locates it under duration and calls it *ellipsis*.) In the first two cases, we have a match between story time and discourse time, but, in the others, we have mismatches. Genette calls the two matches examples of *singulative narration*. Not surprisingly, singulative narration is frequency's default setting, the most common way of handling this aspect of temporality. The first sentence of Tweedy's "People Like Us" provides a good example: "It was a hot, late-summer morning, a month into my first year as a Duke medical student" (11).

Genette calls narrating once something that happens multiple times *iterative narration*. Marcel Proust's opening to *Remembrance of Things Past*, "For a long time I used to go to bed early," is a classic example. Wolff's "Close Calls" provides an especially dramatic instance. Reflecting on how others have died in Vietnam rather than himself, Wolff writes:

> Certainly there were times, not immediately afterward, but in the months and years to come, that I myself had the suspicion it should have been me—that Keith and Hugh and other men had somehow picked up my cards and stood in the place where I was meant to stand.
> (96)

I'll return to Wolff's handling of this "suspicion" when I discuss Wolff's use of fictionality in Chapter 10.

Genette calls narrating multiple times something that happens once *repeating narration*. In "Imelda," the character narrator discovers the event of Franciscus's operation when he sees Imelda's body; he then reports that he imagines it "often" (signaling the iterative) but tells only one version of what he imagines. Then, seeing Imelda's photograph during Franciscus's presentation, he repeats part of what he has visualized: "I could see the long black shadows of her hair flowing into the darker shadows of the morgue."

With duration, Genette focuses on the relation between the length of time an event takes up in the story and the length of time it takes to narrate that event (86–112). Genette acknowledges that, with duration, the border between time and space begins to blur. It's easier to specify how long an event takes up in the story than how long it takes to narrate it, because we can't put a stopwatch on the narrator of a written text. And if we put the stopwatch on readers, we'll find that readers go at different paces. Thus, the metric on the discourse side shifts to a spatial one: how many words, lines, pages are given to the event?

Again, Genette acknowledges multiple possible relations, identifying four main kinds:

1   Scene, in which there's a close match between story time and discourse time. Scene typically involves characters interacting and exchanging dialogue (94–95; 109–112). Tweedy's descriptions of his interactions with Dr. Gale are a good example.
2   Summary, in which the narration of events is briefer than the unfolding of those events (95–99). Oates's "Widow's First Year," with its four-word description of a year's events, is an excellent example. The example of iterative narration from "Close Calls" offers another example, one that illustrates the common link between summary and the iterative.
3   Pause, in which the narration of events is put on hold as the narrator engages in reflections or in exposition of various kinds (99–106). The character narrator's initial description of Honduras in "Imelda" is a good example: "Honduras. I don't suppose I shall ever see it again. Nor do I especially want to. From the plane it seemed a country made of clay—burnt umber, raw sienna, dry." And so on.
4   Ellipsis, in which time passing and events happening in the story are skipped over (106–109). Again "Imelda" provides a good example. After the character narrator delivers his account of how he imagined Franciscus's operation on Imelda in the morgue, Selzer inserts white space and then starts the next paragraph with "Six weeks later." In this case, Selzer sends the signal that the events of the intervening six weeks—the return from Honduras, the resumption of duties, etc.—are not important enough to narrate.[2] In other cases, such as mystery stories, an ellipsis can produce a narrative gap that needs to be filled—either by characters, the

narrator, or readers—in order for the progression to reach a point of resolution. In still other cases, the inability to fill one or more ellipses can have a major function in the narrative. Thomas Pynchon's *The Crying of Lot 49*, with all its unanswered questions about Trystero, the post-horn symbol, and more is a case in point.

Genette mentions a fifth possibility, one in which the narration of events takes longer than the events themselves, but dismisses it as one that rarely occurs. Hannah Courtney has persuasively pushed back, showing that Ian McEwan has frequently made effective use of what she calls a *slowed scene*.[3] In "Sunrise/Sunset," the long narration of Carole's grabbing Jude, bringing him to the terrace, and finally releasing him, with its inclusion of what others are doing as Carole carries Jude, starts as a slowed scene and then shifts into a more standard scene once Jeanne starts talking to Carole.

Genette makes two other remarks that add appropriate nuance to this analysis of time. The first is that, as we have already seen with ellipsis as something that could be included as a type of either frequency or duration, the aspects of temporality are not walled off from each other but rather often overlap. To take another example, summary (from the duration group) often relies on iterative narration (from the frequency group). The second point is that the relations between story time and discourse time can't always be discerned clearly. Sometimes the narration does not allow readers to infer chronological order, or how many times something happened, or how long it took for them to happen. When there is such lack of clarity about these matters, we have what David Herman has aptly called "fuzzy temporality."

In addition to drawing on Genette's work, rhetorical theory finds considerable value in Mikhail Bakhtin's interest in the interaction of time and space in narrative, a phenomenon he labels the *chronotope*. Bakhtin defines the term this way:

> In the literary artistic chronotope, spatial and temporal indicators are fused into one carefully thought-out, concrete whole. Time, as it were, thickens, takes on flesh, becomes artistically visible; likewise, space becomes charged and responsive to the movements of time, plot and history.
>
> (84)

For Bakhtin, the concept helps us grasp core features of some genres such as the novel of the road. Shlomith Rimmon-Kenan and Susan S. Lanser have used Bakhtin's concept to great effect in their essay, "Narratology at the Checkpoint," which analyzes narratives addressing issues along the Israel-Palestine border. In the next chapter on space, I'll consider how the concept of the chronotope can give us further insight into Oates's "Hospice/Honeymoon."

Rhetorical theory integrates this work on temporality by situating it within its ruling idea that authors construct narratives by shaping raw materials in order to achieve particular effects in relation to target audiences. In practice, this integration works by shifting away from strict comparisons between story time and discourse time to the more flexible idea that authors shape both the temporality of events and the temporality of narration in constructing their purposive narrative progressions. Furthermore, rhetorical theory then takes the additional step of attending to the interactions of the shaping of temporality and other resources and to the multi-layered effects of such shaping on rhetorical readers. I will seek to clarify these points in the analysis of temporality and perspective in Danticat's "Sunrise/Sunset" and of temporality and the progression of lyric narrative in "This Old Man."

Before I begin that analysis, I'd like to step back from the detailed explanations of order, frequency, and duration to show that attending to the way the primary narratives of the texts in our corpus (some to be discussed in upcoming chapters) depict change over time provides helpful insights into each.

1   Angell, "This Old Man." Primary (lyric) narrative: Revelation of his situation and his assessment of it through his half-hour (or so) address to his narratee/authorial audience.
2   Chast, *Can't We Talk about Something More Pleasant?* Primary narrative: The final years of Chast's parents' lives.
3   Danticat, "Sunrise/Sunset." Primary narrative: Carole's movement further into dementia and Jeanne's movement away from post-partum depression during a few hours of Jude's christening day.
4   Miriam Engelberg, *Cancer Made Me a Shallower Person.* Primary narrative: Engelberg's experiences of diagnosis, treatment, and recurrence of breast cancer over an indefinite but relatively short period.
5   Gilman, "The Yellow Wallpaper." Primary narrative: The character narrator's transformation over a few months of captivity (aka rest cure) into someone who has lost her grip on reality.
6   Oates, "Hospice/Honeymoon." Primary narrative: The climactic moments of the protagonist's movement from denial to acceptance of her husband's need for hospice care.
7   Oates, "Widow's First Year." Primary narrative: The protagonist's year-long, successful struggle to survive.
8   Selzer, "Imelda." Primary narrative: Franciscus's positive change in character as a result of two days with Imelda and her mother and their aftermath.
9   Tweedy, "People Like Us." Primary narrative: Tweedy the character proving to himself by proving to Dr. Gale over the course of his first semester that he belongs at Duke.
10 Tóibín, "One Minus One." Primary (portrait) narrative: Revelation of the protagonist's character during the course of his imaginary half-hour (or so) phone call.

11   Jesmyn Ward, "On Witness and Respair." Primary narrative: Ward's developing responses to the two main events in her life from January to August 2020, the death of her husband from COVID-19 and the Black Lives Matter protests after the killing of George Floyd.

12   Wolff, "Close Calls." Primary narrative: Wolff's three experiences of almost being killed during his year-long tour of duty in Vietnam.

Time and Perspective in Danticat's "Sunrise, Sunset"

As I noted briefly in the discussion of Danticat's story in Chapter 3, she includes a backstory, which we can now call an analepsis, about Carole's childhood in Haiti. Taking a closer look can not only offer further insight into Danticat's story but also illustrate how time and perspective often work together. Danticat does not do anything to set up the analepsis but instead suddenly shifts into it, as she also shifts from Jeanne's perspective to the narrator's:

> Carole and her childhood friend Jeanne used to talk to each other through a hole they'd poked in the plywood that separated their rooms. In the morning, when Jeanne went to fetch water at the neighborhood tap, she would whistle a wake-up call to Carole. Jeanne's whistle sounded like the squeaky chirping of a pipirit gri, the gray kingbirds that flew around the area until boys knocked them down with slingshots, roasted them in firepits, and ate them.
>
> One morning, Jeanne did not whistle, and Carole never saw her again ….
>
> The next occupant of that room was Victor …. Victor soon discovered the hole in the plywood and would slip his finger through and wave it at her. Then she would whistle to him, like the last kingbird of their neighborhood.

What stands out first is how economical the analepsis is, that is, how much information about Carole's past Danticat packs into a few short paragraphs. She achieves this economy by relying almost exclusively on iterative narration. Indeed, she uses singulative narration only once to report that "One morning Jeanne did not whistle," and she follows that report with the summary: "and Carole never saw her again." By keeping the duration short, Danticat also keeps the dominant focus of the story on the action of the primary narrative, the differing trajectories of Carole and her daughter Jeanne on Jude's christening day, which she reports in the present tense. Nevertheless, Danticat uses the analepsis to create multiple important effects.

Although Danticat does not explicitly mark the reach of the analepsis, rhetorical readers can readily infer that it must be more than 40 years. Similarly, Danticat does not clearly reveal the extent of the analepsis across all that iterative narration, but rhetorical readers can recognize that it goes from Carole's childhood to the time she and Victor immigrated to Miami. I noted previously that two effects of the analepsis are to further contextualize Carole's current situation, especially her differences from her daughter, born in the USA, and to bring in another layer to the metaphor of sunrise/sunset that frames the whole story. A closer look reveals additional effects: (a) it emphasizes Carole's status as an immigrant to the US, the way in which her life can be divided into two time periods—life in Haiti and life in the US; (b) despite leaving Haiti, Carole affirmed her attachment to the place by naming her daughter after her childhood friend, and thus bringing her past into her present; (c) Carole and Victor's relationship, because it is so similar to Carole's with her childhood friend, is built on friendship. Indeed, Danticat's analepsis presents Victor as a substitute for Jeanne, even as it emphasizes Carole's exercise of her agency in courting Victor: she replaces Jeanne as the one who whistles like the kingbirds; (d) Carole grew up in poverty: the wall between her room and Jeanne's room was so thin that they could poke a hole in it with their fingers; the boys were so hungry that they shot down the kingbirds and then roasted and ate them; and by the time Carole and Victor were communicating through the hole in the wall, Carole was whistling like "the last" kingbird.

These effects have multiple consequences for readerly dynamics. They deepen rhetorical readers' alignment with Carole by giving a fuller sense of her life course, including its struggles and joys—all before the onset of her dementia. Indeed, the analepsis allows rhetorical readers to see aspects of Carole's life that Jeanne apparently has not, and, in so doing, increases those readers' understanding of the gaps between the two characters that are exacerbated by their current conditions. This understanding in turn makes the rapprochement that the story ends with all the more moving.

Danticat concludes the analepsis by shifting to Carole's perspective at the time of the past action: "Carole knew from the moment she met Victor that he would take care of her." But then, just as Danticat abruptly shifted into the analepsis, she shifts back to the present—and to the perspective of the now cognitively impaired Carole: "She never thought he'd conspire against her, or even threaten to put her away. But here he is now, plotting against her with a woman she does not know, a fleshy, pretty woman, just the way he once liked them, just the way she was, when he liked her most." The effects of the analepsis make these temporal and perspectival shifts almost heartbreaking: Carole totally misevaluates Victor and she fails to recognize her own daughter, even as she perceives Jeanne's resemblance to her younger self.

Furthermore, as Danticat continues with the present-tense action she shows how Carole's present cognition is mixed up with her memories of Haiti. Mistaking Jeanne's baby Jude for the doll Victor has given her to practice with before his birth, Carole thinks: "why is she sitting next to this peppercorn-haired doll that her husband sometimes uses to trick her, pretending it's a real baby. Her real babies are gone. They disappeared with her friend Jeanne, and all she has left is this doll her husband bought her." Then, recognizing that the "doll" seems upset, she seeks to calm him down by whistling "the pipirit's spirited squeak."

Danticat's bringing the past into the present in this way adds considerable depth and texture to her own remarkable perspective-taking in the story. Carole's cognitive decline is undeniable but far from random. It has connections to her past experiences, to her love for her husband and her daughter, and to so much that has made her who she is.

Time and Lyric Narrative in "This Old Man"

I choose Angell's text for the deeper dive because its concern with old age is inextricably tied to issues of temporality. Indeed, it provides further evidence for my claim that time and narrative are transcultural because every culture needs to come to terms with birth and death. Not surprisingly, Angell is far more concerned with the latter than the former. I also choose Angell's text because his handling of its lyric narrative form makes it a tour de force demonstration of the interrelations among lyric, narrative, and time as well as the mimetic and thematic components of character. As a lyric narrative, concerned with "the way I and others my age live now," the dominant tense is the present, but virtually every paragraph is chock full of salient uses of temporality. I won't of course analyze them all but instead will focus on a few that I find especially remarkable and relevant to an understanding of the whole piece. I start with a fuller account of its lyric narrative progression.

Angell's first and last sentences give a general picture of its movement, as he starts with "Check me out" and ends with "Take it from us, who know about the emptiness of loss, and are still cruising along here feeling lucky and not yet entirely alone." In both sentences he uses a present-tense direct address to an uncharacterized narratee. But the shift from "me" to "us" indicates another movement, an expansion beyond the mimetic focus on himself to a thematic concern for others like himself. By linking his current situation (itself informed by his past experiences) to the situations of other old people, he moves from portraiture to lyric as the dominant mode of the progression. In this way, Angell works with his own version of the mimetic-thematic feedback loop: his self-portrait is an important basis for his reflections on commonalities among the aging, even as those broader reflections give additional significance to that self-portrait. In addition, the last sentence functions as a rough summary of the lyric situation, one in which he and others are marked by the experience of loss but not overpowered by it, and thus still desire human connection.

Angell takes his time (!) getting to this last sentence, and, indeed, one of the pleasures of the progression is its temporal unfolding. He takes up and reflects upon, in this order, the following dimensions of his situation:

- his physical condition
- his experiences of loss
- the consolations of memory and the frustrations of its imperfections
- the support of family and friends
- sources of pleasure and happiness
- the feeling of being invisible to younger people
- thoughts about death
- his intellectual activities
- his reliance on and pleasure in jokes
- his ongoing needs for deep attachment and intimate love
- his concluding recommendations about old people meeting those needs.

Angell makes sometimes abrupt and sometimes smooth segues from one dimension to another. For example, he moves from his physical condition to his thoughts about death by saying "Let's move on," but he links his reflections on jokes about sex to his reflections on the need for intimacy. Furthermore, because the overall progression is not one of instability—complication—resolution, Angell has some leeway with his arrangement of the issues he takes up. It doesn't greatly matter whether he discusses his intellectual activities or the support of family friends in the first half or the second half of the piece. But the arrangement is far from random. It makes sense to start with his physical condition and to end with his recommendations. It also makes sense to take up loss and death in the beginning and the middle of the progression in order to make them key parts of his lyric exploration without having them undermine the more positive affirmation of life and connection at the end. Finally, it makes sense to move back and forth between positive and negative aspects of his situation in order to better convey its mixture of problems and pleasures.

This summary gets at the overarching logic of Angell's construction, but its power depends on the texture of his reflections, and that texture depends in large part on his handling of temporality. Here are a few examples.

> I'm ninety-three, and I'm feeling great. Well, pretty great, unless I've forgotten to take a couple of Tylenols in the past four or five hours, in which case I've begun to feel some jagged little pains shooting down my left forearm and into the base of the thumb. Shingles, in 1996, with resultant nerve damage.

Angell starts with a present-tense claim that initially appears to be singulative and positive. But the qualification converts it to a singulative occurrence within the broader implied iterative accompanying his age: "I'm ninety-three and how I'm feeling all depends." Furthermore, in spelling out what his feeling depends on, he uses one analepsis with a short reach and short extent ("a couple of Tylenols in the past four or five hours") that soon takes him into another one with a longer reach and a longer extent ("Shingles, in 1996"). It's not just that he's almost giving rhetorical readers whiplash as he speeds from present to recent past to less recent past but also that he's linking how he's feeling to both past events. The takeaway is that "how I feel now has far less to do with now than with the past." Finally, the rapid temporal movement gives energy to Angell's voice—he's in command and moving rapidly—and that effect increases its appeal.

Now consider this later passage from the section on his physical condition:

> The lower-middle sector of my spine twists and jogs like a Connecticut county road, thanks to a herniated disk seven or eight years ago. This has cost me two or three inches of height, transforming me from Gary Cooper to Geppetto. After days spent groaning on the floor, I received a blessed epidural, ending the ordeal. "You can sit up now," the doctor said, whisking off his shower cap. "Listen, do you know who Dominic Chianese is?"
>
> "Isn't that Uncle Junior?" I said, confused. "You know—from 'The Sopranos'?"
>
> "Yes," he said. "He and I play in a mandolin quartet every Wednesday night at the Hotel Edison. Do you think you could help us get a listing in the front of *The New Yorker*?"

Here Angell rings some changes on his strategy of moving rapidly back and forth between present and past. He starts with the present ("twists and jogs" now), then moves to past ("herniated disk seven or eight years ago"), then back to present ("has cost me"—note the hint of the iterative), and then back to the past, first for the iterative narration of "days groaning on the floor" and then finally arrives at the theater-of-the-incongruous scene with the doctor. That sudden stop at what, in this context, is a longish scene enhances its absurd humor. Look at this juxtaposition, Angell seems to say. Combined with the freshness of the prose itself (note the metaphor of his uneven spine as a Connecticut county road), Angell's handling of temporality contributes to his communication of his pleasure in still being alive.

But it's far from all pleasure. One of the most moving paragraphs comes in the section on loss.

> Here in my tenth decade, I can testify that the downside of great age is the room it provides for rotten news. Living long means enough already. When [our dog] Harry died [three years ago], Carol and I couldn't stop weeping; we sat in the bathroom with his retrieved body on a mat between us, the light-brown patches on his back and the near-black of his ears still darkened by the rain, and passed a Kleenex box back and forth between us. Not all the tears were for him. Two months earlier, a beautiful daughter of mine, my oldest child, had ended her life, and the oceanic force and mystery of that event had not

left full space for tears. Now we could cry without reserve, weep together for Harry and Callie and ourselves. Harry cut us loose.

Rather than moving back and forth between present and past here, Angell moves from present to past and stays in the past. The duration of the passage is longer than usual in this piece, and that duration is connected to Angell's ability to express how clock time gives way to experiential time: although the deaths of his dog and his daughter are separated by two months of clock time, his tears for Callie have remained suppressed until he cries for Harry. In this connection, the "Now" in "Now we could cry without reserve" still refers to the past ("could cry" rather than "can cry"), but it works to bring the two events together. This layering of events in combination with the duration of time allows Angell to suggest that the "oceanic" force of Callie's suicide is now felt in a corresponding ocean of tears. But as he ends with summary, Angell characteristically turns toward the positive: "Harry cut us loose." Harry, in other words, has done them one more service. Their tears have been cathartic.

Angell doesn't wait until the last paragraph to thematize his experiences. In the next paragraph, he writes:

> A few notes about age is my aim here, but a little more about loss is inevitable. "Most of the people my age is dead. You could look it up" was the way Casey Stengel put it. He was seventy-five at the time, and contemporary social scientists might prefer Casey's line delivered at eighty-five now, for accuracy, but the point remains. We geezers carry about a bulging directory of dead husbands or wives, children, parents, lovers, brothers and sisters, dentists and shrinks, office sidekicks, summer neighbors, classmates, and bosses, all once entirely familiar to us and seen as part of the safe landscape of the day. It's no wonder we're a bit bent. The surprise, for me, is that the accruing weight of these departures doesn't bury us, and that even the pain of an almost unbearable loss gives way quite quickly to something more distant but still stubbornly gleaming. The dead have departed, but gestures and glances and tones of voice of theirs, even scraps of clothing—that pale-yellow Saks scarf—reappear unexpectedly, along with accompanying touches of sweetness or irritation.

Angell again moves from present to past (when he quotes that famous philosopher Casey Stengel), but when he returns to the present and shifts to the first-person plural, he does something different. His dominant tense is the present, but in the middle of the paragraph it becomes what I'll call a *layered present* because it's imbued with the past: once he mentions the contents of that "bulging directory," he—and his rhetorical readers—can't help but look back. Angell's looking back finally takes him to the actual past, though signaled not by a past-tense verb but by the temporal adverb "once," to the time when the dead were "once entirely familiar ... and seen as part of the safe landscape of the day." The final sentence offers another variation on the layered present as the unexpected reappearances of the dead inevitably call to mind the past. Angell accompanies the layered present with the merging of the individual and the general, as the move from "the surprise, for me," to "these departures don't bury us" indicates. Even more arresting in this merging of past and present is his move from the general to the specific, from the category "scraps of clothing" to that evocative particular "pale-yellow Saks scarf." The paragraph's method and effects call to mind Oates's "Widow's First Year": there's so much going on beneath the surface here.

Angell ends the piece with his discussion of the biggest surprise of his life, "our unceasing need for deep attachment and intimate love," which is arguably the most important dimension of his current condition:

> Here's to you, old dears. You got this right, every one of you. Hook, line, and sinker; never mind the why or wherefore; somewhere in the night; love me forever, or at least until next week. For us and for anyone this unsettles, anyone who's younger and still squirms at the vision of an old couple embracing, I'd offer John Updike's "Sex or death: you take your pick"—a line that appears (in a slightly different form) in a late story of his, "Playing with Dynamite."
>
> This is a great question, an excellent insurance-plan choice, I mean. I think it's in the Affordable Care Act somewhere. Take it from us, who know about the emptiness of loss, and are still cruising along here feeling lucky and not yet entirely alone.

Not surprisingly, Angell stays in the present tense, even as he varies his narratees: he starts by addressing "old dears"; shifts to the unnamed other being asked to "love me forever"; and ends with everyone (except those included in the "us" of the last sentence). That variation is part and parcel of what he's doing with duration here, which in turn connects with what he's doing with lyric and narrative. Rather than offering a final scene or even a slowed scene to complete a narrative of change, Angell lingers over the crucial insight into the condition of old age. Rather than reporting or dramatizing action, Angell focuses on his thematic takeaway, playing it out, joking about and with it, and then ending with the ultimately serious line that encapsulates so much of what he's previously explored: "the emptiness of loss [while still] feeling lucky and not yet entirely alone."

Opening Out

The concluding phrase in the rhetorical definition of narrative, "something happened," can be paraphrased as "something changed over time." All storytellers, whether working with narratives that conform readily to the default definition or with hybrid forms such as portrait narratives, lyric narratives, and essay narratives, have multiple ways of handling temporality at their disposal. Caregivers who attend carefully to how patients handle time in telling about their conditions can learn about what matters most to them. Listening for departures from standard chronology, for shifts from the time of the action to the time of the telling, and for repetitions (frequency), emphases, and ellipses (duration) can reveal a lot about both the teller's primary concerns and their affective relation to those concerns. Caregivers should also be open to the ways in which patients prioritize subjective time over clock or calendar time rather than automatically viewing it as evidence of deficient narration. Patients, for their part, can attend to how caregivers handle time in their treatment recommendations: do they refer to past experiences? Do they predict likely outcomes? What aspects do they emphasize and what do they minimize by their handling of frequency and duration?

Overstanding Prompt

Respond to this claim: "My Old Man" is undermined by Angell's lack of awareness of his own privilege as a white heterosexual male in twenty-first century USA; he has had and still has advantages in life that make it impossible for his thematizing of his age to be persuasive to anyone who is not so privileged. Make the case for this position and then respond to it, agreeing or disagreeing, in whole or in part, and giving warrants for your response.

Springboarding Prompts

Using Angell's piece as a model, write a lyric narrative with similar mimetic–thematic relationships, that is, use your self-representation as the basis for some broader thematizing about the group(s) you identify yourself as a member of. Feel free to play off Angell's title, by, for instance, using "This Young Feminist," "This Queer Rebel," and so on.

Write a story about characters whose interactions are significantly influenced by a large gap in their ages.

Write a story that highlights the difference between clock time and subjective time.

Write a story about an experience that prompted you to understand your age in a new way.

Notes

1 Paul Ricœur, *Time and Narrative*, 3.
2 Robyn Warhol would call this ellipsis an instance of the "subnarratable." See her insightful discussion about what doesn't get told in "Neonarrative."
3 Courtney, Hannah. "Narrative Temporality and Slowed Scene: The Interaction of Event and Thought Representation in Ian McEwan's Fiction."

Works Cited

Angell, Roger. "This Old Man." *The New Yorker*, 9 February 2014. www.new yorker.com/magazine/2014/02/17/old-man-3 (Accessed 13 December 2021.)

Bakhtin, M.M. *The Dialogic Imagination*, edited by Michael Holquist, translated by Caryl Emerson and Michael Holquist. Austin, TX: University of Texas Press, 1981.

Cohn, Dorrit. *The Distinction of Fiction*. Baltimore, MD: Johns Hopkins University Press, 1999.

Courtney, Hannah. "Narrative Temporality and Slowed Scene: The Interaction of Event and Thought Representation in Ian McEwan's Fiction." *Narrative* 21, 2 (2013): 180–197.

Danticat, Edwidge. "Sunrise/Sunset." *The New Yorker*, 11 September 2017. www.new yorker.com/magazine/2017/09/18/sunrise-sunset (Accessed 10 February 2022.)

Genette, Gérard. *Narrative Discourse: An Essay in Method*, translated by Jane E. Lewin. Ithaca, NY: Cornell University Press, 1980.

Herman, David. *Story Logic: Problems and Possibilities of Narrative*. Lincoln, NE: University of Nebraska Press, 2002.

Lanser, Susan S. and Shlomith Rimmon-Kenan. "Narratology at the Checkpoint: The Politics and Poetics of Entanglement." *Narrative* 27 (2019): 245–269.

Ricœur, Paul. *Time and Narrative*, Vol. 1, translated by Kathleen McLaughlin and David Pellauer. Chicago, IL: University of Chicago Press, 1984.

Selzer, Richard. "Imelda." In *The Doctor Stories*, 83–97. New York: Picador, 1998.

Tweedy, Damon. *Black Man in a White Coat: A Doctor's Reflections on Race and Medicine*. London: Picador, 2015.

Warhol, Robyn. "Neonarrative: Or, How to Narrate the Unnarratable in Realist Fiction and Contemporary Film." In *A Companion to Narrative Theory*, edited by James Phelan and Peter J. Rabinowitz, 220–231. Oxford: Wiley-Blackwell, 2005.

8 Space

For a long time, narrative theory didn't devote a lot of attention (time or space!) to space. Happily, the situation is now different, and the reasons for both the relative neglect and the increased attention are instructive. Given that most narrative theorists include the idea of "change over time" in their conceptions of narrative, they initially found it natural to privilege time over space as they theorized narrative. Such accounts included space but typically relegated it to the background of both narrative and theory, by merging it with (some aspects of) time in the concept of setting. Gérard Genette's concept of "pause," which describes a situation in which the narration stops focusing on the forward movement of action in time and focuses instead on narratorial musings or on descriptions of various types, including those about space, reflects the older tendency to privilege time over space. To put it paradoxically, setting is not where the (theoretical) action was. The situation has changed for multiple reasons, but the most important reflect the interaction between narrative practice and narrative theory.

First, in looking at narrative practice, theorists recognized that storytellers frequently make space more than just background for the action. Sometimes authors give space an importance similar to that of characters, as William Faulkner does with his fictional Yoknapatawpha County, Mississippi, and as Zora Neale Hurston does with the nonfictional Eatonville, Florida in her novel *Their Eyes Were Watching God*. Sometimes, authors use characters' movement from one space to another to signal other kinds of change. In *The Underground Railroad*, Colson Whitehead tracks the movement of his protagonist Cora across various states in the southern United States in the 1850s. Whitehead represents each state as providing its distinctive threats to Cora's quest for freedom, because each has its own way of implementing its white supremacist ideology. In addition, certain changes of space such as the "descent into the underworld" become tropes that signify across narratives (e.g., the descent is often a revelation of the unconscious or a test of moral and physical strength) even as authors can adapt them for their own purposes. But even when space doesn't become so prominent, it frequently becomes more than just background for action. Some authors show how it looms large in characters' perceptions and desires, as Oates does in "Hospice/Honeymoon."

DOI: 10.4324/9781003018865-8

Second, as narrative theorists became increasingly interested in developing as comprehensive accounts of narrative as possible, they recognized the need to correct the privileging of time over space and to move beyond limiting considerations of space to setting. Marie-Laure Ryan has offered a helpful taxonomy of spatial concepts in this vein.[1] Her taxonomy moves from more specific to more general delineations:

1   Spatial frames: the places in which events occur such as rooms, build-ings, streets, parks, and so on. "The Yellow Wallpaper" stands out among our narratives not only because it is largely confined to the single spatial frame of the house in which the protagonist undergoes her rest cure but also because the protagonist's relation to one aspect of that frame—the wallpaper in her bedroom—dominates the narrative.

2   Story space: the sum total of the spatial frames of the narrative. In "One Minus One," for example, the story space includes Texas, New York, and various places in Ireland.

3   Setting: the spatial-temporal context for the narrative, e.g., Little Haiti in Miami, Florida in the early twenty-first century for "Sunrise/Sunset."

4   Storyworld: the larger world containing the story space, completed by the reader's imagination as informed by relevant cultural knowledge. Thus, in "Imelda," the main story spaces are the US medical school where Franciscus teaches and Honduras, but the storyworld consists of the Western Hemisphere. In discussing how readers fill out storyworlds in fiction, Ryan has helpfully proposed the "principle of minimal departure," which stipulates that the fictional world corresponds to the actual world unless the narrative specifies otherwise. Thus, a teller who constructs a storyworld without an explicit reference to, say, the law of gravity, will expect their readers to assume that the law holds in that storyworld. More generally, the principle means that readers can fill out minimally described storyworlds with features of the actual world.

5   Narrative universe: the actual world constructed by the text plus all the other worlds projected or imagined by narrators or characters. In "Hospice/Honeymoon" the narrative universe includes not only the actual spaces of hospital and home but also the protagonist's imagi-native projection of her home as a space in which hospice could become honeymoon.

Ryan locates her work in the broader field of cognitive narratology because it is concerned with the relation between the spaces (and possible worlds) of the text and readers' mental activity in constructing or reconstructing those spaces. David Herman, another cognitive narratologist, has proposed making the concept of storyworld and the activity of world-building central to the understanding of narrative. Rhetorical theory sees great value in this cognitive work on space, but characteristically modifies it. In line with the Author—Resources—Audience model, rhetorical theory sees space and world-building as central to some narratives and less central to others. For example, Oates's "Widow's First Year" does not foreground issues of space and neither do many other short narratives. But it's not just a matter of length. Authors of most portrait narratives and lyric narratives are less concerned with constructing storyworlds than with revealing character and situation respectively. Actual readers can certainly fill out larger storyworlds in these narratives, but, as we've seen with Tóibín's "One Minus One" and Angell's "This Old Man," that activity is not as crucial to understanding Tóibín's and Angell's purposes as understanding what they do with the resources of character and time. Refining things further, I would say that the spatial frames and storyworld of Tóibín's portrait are more central than those of Angell's lyric narrative. By contrast, Oates in "Hospice/Honeymoon" and Gilman in "The Yellow Wallpaper," as I'll discuss later in this chapter, give greater emphasis to the spatial frames and the storyworlds of their narratives than Tóibín or Angell do in theirs.

Rhetorical theory also recognizes that authorial uses of space in narrative frequently rely on broader ideas about space in culture. Space in culture is a relational entity: any one space is typically part of some constellation of spaces in which the significance of each is at least partially determined by its relation to others. Thus, for example, the meaning of an examination room in a medical office depends in part on its difference from the waiting room, on the one hand, and a doctor's private office, on the other. The same relationality typically operates in narrative. In *The Underground Railroad*, Georgia with its cotton plantations and direct oppression of enslaved people, South Carolina with its superficially enlightened attitudes and insidious covert oppressions, and North Carolina with its overt celebrations of lynchings form an especially powerful constellation of similarity-within-difference, a constellation given further shape by the additional spatial frames of Tennessee, Indiana, and The North.

More generally, culture has defined certain spaces and their relationality in particular ways. For example, domestic space is different from space in the public sphere, and acts in one (e.g., expressions of sexual intimacy) are often not appropriate in the other. Similarly, underground space exists in opposition to above ground space. Again, authors of both fiction and nonfiction work with these culturally accepted relations of space and adapt them for their own purposes.

Moving to more fine-grained analyses of the representations of space in narrative, rhetorical theory also finds it helpful to draw on work from other traditions of narrative theory. Franz Stanzel has suggested a distinction between aperspectival and perspectival representations. As the terms suggest, aperspectival representations are not tied to a view from a fixed position or character, while perspectival ones are. The analepsis in Danticat's "Sunrise/Sunset" provides a good example:

> Carole and her childhood friend Jeanne used to talk to each other through a hole they'd poked in the plywood that separated their rooms. In the morning, when Jeanne went to fetch water at the

neighborhood tap, she would whistle a wake-up call to Carole. Jeanne's whistle sounded like the squeaky chirping of a pipirit gri, the gray kingbirds that flew around the area until boys knocked them down with slingshots, roasted them in firepits, and ate them.

Danticat's narrator informs the narratee about various aspects of Carole's spatial environment in Haiti—the rooms of Carole and Jeanne, the external water tap, the sky that was sometimes full of kingbirds, the fire pits in which boys roasted them. But the orientation is not tied to Carole's perspective and the narrator is not tied to any single location. This technique allows Danticat to communicate reliably and efficiently, desirable effects because she wants to subordinate this backstory about Carole's childhood to the events in the unfolding primary narrative. As we have seen, Danticat anchors the rest of the story in the perspectives of Carole and her daughter Jeanne (named for Carole's childhood friend).

Now compare that passage with Tobias Wolff's account of his first close call.

> I sat up and looked around. The crowd had drawn back in a wide circle. They were staring at me. A woman yammered something I couldn't follow and pointed under the jeep. I bent down for a look. There, lying directly below my seat was a hand grenade. The pin had been pulled.
>
> (90)

This passage is strikingly different from Danticat's not only in its content but in its perspectival approach to space. Wolff locates the experiencing-I in his jeep in the town square of his village in Vietnam and has him represent the space and the action from that fixed location: I was here, the crowd was there, the grenade was right below me. This perspective of course heightens rhetorical readers' sense of the danger in the scene.

Marie-Laure Ryan has helpfully pointed out two common ways of representing space from either the aperspectival or the perspectival position: the map and the tour (Ryan, *Narrating Space*). The map provides an atemporal snapshot of a space that also indicates where entities are located in relation to each other. The tour, on the other hand, connects space to time in the sense that it lends itself to motion-through-space, as in "starting here, you see X, and then moving there, you see Y." In "The Yellow Wallpaper," Gilman has the character narrator, located in her bedroom, offer a partial perspectival tour of the area outside the house:

> Out of one window I can see the garden, those mysterious deep-shaded arbors, the riotous old-fashioned flowers, and bushes and gnarly trees.
>
> Out of another I get a lovely view of the bay and a little private wharf belonging to the estate. There is a beautiful shaded lane that runs down there from the house.
>
> (1394)

Not surprisingly, rhetorical theory finds it productive to think about the functions of space in relation to the three components of narrative construction and readerly interest: the mimetic, thematic, and synthetic. With space, the mimetic function involves the depiction of actual or plausible spaces, the thematic involves the ideational dimensions of particular spaces, and the synthetic involves (a) the author's depictions of anti-mimetic, that is, impossible or extreme, and thus obviously constructed spaces, and (b) the functions of space in the construction of their narrative. Thus, for example, Gilman shows how the character narrator moves from her initial description of a mimetically plausible bedroom to later descriptions of an impossible one. But that movement remains within the realm of the mimetic, since it follows from the plausible way the character narrator changes under the stress of her enforced rest cure. Gilman, then, links this mimetic dimension of her representation of the space to the thematic function of representing consequences of patriarchal oppression. If, however, Gilman had signaled that the character narrator's telling was wholly reliable, then Gilman would be working with a synthetic, impossible space and doing a different kind of thematizing of it. I'll elaborate on this point below. For now, let's consider two other examples.

In "Imelda," Selzer uses a perspectival tour as his character narrator describes the space around the hospital in Comayagua, Honduras, and by melding the description of the space with the description of the people who occupy it, Selzer thematizes it:

> Just in front of the hospital was a thirsty courtyard where mobs of waiting people squatted or lay in the meager shade ... . Against the walls of this courtyard, gaunt, dejected men stood, their faces, like their country, preternaturally solemn, leaden.
>
> (24)

Franciscus, then, encounters Imelda in a space saturated with the leaden weight of dejection, and this space contributes to all the dynamics at work in the encounter between doctor and patient. As noted in Chapter 3, Selzer's attitudes about Honduras as a "third-world" country that underlie this thematizing can provide grounds for a negative overstanding of his story.

In "Sunrise/Sunset," Danticat offers an example of how the mimetic function of space simultaneously serves a synthetic function. Toward the end of the story, the narration from Carole's perspective reveals that "They [the EMTs] are about to roll her out of the apartment." This development is the mimetically plausible culmination of the sequence of events on Jude's christening day. But Danticat also uses Carole's perception about her imminent removal from the apartment to signal to her audience that this phase of Carole's life—and, indeed, the story itself—is ending. Danticat reinforces these synthetic effects by tracing Carole's perceptions that her daughter may be playing the "Sunrise/Sunset" game with her.

As I now turn to analyze space in "Hospice/Honeymoon" and "The Yellow Wallpaper," I will draw on these theoretical accounts but give the greatest emphasis to the mimetic, thematic, and synthetic functions that follow from Oates's and Gilman's deployments of space.

Chronotopes and Spatial Frames in "Hospice/Honeymoon"

As I noted in the previous chapter, Mikhail Bakhtin's concept of the chronotope can illuminate Oates's work with both time and space in "Hospice/Honeymoon." As you'll recall, Bakhtin notes that in the chronotope, "spatial and temporal indicators are fused into one carefully thought-out, concrete whole. Time, as it were, thickens, takes on flesh, becomes artistically visible; likewise, space becomes charged and responsive to the movements of time, plot and history" (84). Both hospice and honeymoon qualify as chronotopes, since both rely on the fusing of time and space. Oates reinforces their chronotopic quality with her narration. As the narrator addresses the protagonist, she uses an extended spatial-temporal metaphor to describe hospice: "the *vast Sahara* that lies ahead with all that you cannot bear, *that nonetheless will be borne,* and by you" (my emphasis). The protagonist describes honeymoon by envisioning spaces in the house in iterative terms. In the rented hospital bed, "*I will sleep beside my husband holding him in my arms.*" The fusions of space and time in each chronotope are radically different as reflected in each one's thematic meanings. Hospice evokes a difficult space-time that puts burdens on both an individual in their final days and their loved ones, and honeymoon conjures an idyllic space-time shared by a couple at the start of a marriage.

More generally, Oates uses the synthetic device of contrasting chronotopes to add significant layers to the mimetic and thematic components of her story. At the mimetic level, the contrast indicates just how deeply the protagonist is in denial: unable to face the reality of one chronotope, she tries to speak the other into existence. At the thematic level, Oates uses the chronotopes to set the protagonist's responses within larger, readily legible systems of meaning to make them plausibly representative of other women—indeed, other people—trying to come to terms with a beloved partner's final days.

Turning to the spatial frames, we can readily identify two: the hospital, where the protagonist's husband is being treated for cancer, and their imaginatively transformed home. (The story has a third, indeterminate space, the location in which the exchange between narrator and protagonist occurs, but that indeterminacy suggests that Oates is far less concerned with the space itself than with the tellings that occur within it.)

At first glance, Oates may seem to be using the hospital as a necessary but insignificant backdrop for her representation of the main action, the progression of the protagonist's attitudes about her husband's "final days." She has the narrator mention the hospital only once, and that mention is itself in the background. The narrator reports that the protagonist's husband first utters the word "hospice," "On the phone very early one morning, when he calls, as he has been calling, immediately after the oncologist making rounds in the hospital has examined him." In the narrator's next sentence, Oates indicates that it is less the hospital itself that matters for this utterance than the physical separation between the couple: "On the phone, so that he is spared seeing your face. And you, his." The couple need the physical distance because they are so emotionally and psychologically far apart in their ability to accept that he is entering his final days. But as the story progresses, Oates indicates that the actual space of the hospital influences the protagonist's imagined transformation of her home. She wants to create a space for her husband that is, in her own words *"NOT the Cancer Center."* Instead, *"Our hospice will be in our home, which he loves."* Behind the protagonist's statement is her recognition of the difference between the hospital as a public, or at least non-domestic, space controlled by the medical staff, and home as a private, domestic space that she can arrange as she likes.

The protagonist's imagined space is obviously an idealized version of their home, one that she fills out by envisioning how she can link aspects of the home to pleasing, as much as possible, four of her husband's five senses— seeing, touching, hearing, and tasting—and his presumed interest in a social life. In other words, she imagines the space as especially appealing in ways that are either not possible or far more difficult to achieve in the hospital and that collectively deny the notion of final days. Oates uses the contrast between the spatial frames to add further texture to the mimetic-thematic feedback loop.

Although the final twist of the story depends not on Oates's handling of space but on her handling of the attunement between narrator and protagonist, the previous work with space gives the final lines greater weight. *"Hospice,* yes. *Honeymoon,* no" is not just a necessary reality check and adjustment, but also a recognition and acceptance by the protagonist of what her experience of the hospice chronotope is likely to be.

Space and Bonding Unreliability in "The Yellow Wallpaper"

Theorists who equate the construction of a narrative with a construction of a storyworld make the sound point that many narratives ask their readers to add details to flesh out the world. Marie-Laure Ryan's principle of minimal departure helps capture how that filling out works. As noted earlier, rhetorical theory endorses the principle, but finds it more relevant for some narratives than others. Gilman's "The Yellow Wallpaper" is a case in which constructing and re-constructing a storyworld is central to understanding its nexus of author—audience—purposes. Gilman invites her rhetorical readers to recognize that the character narrator's experience in the spatial frame of her rented house and the slightly larger story space (the area surrounding the house and the environment she is getting away from) directly follows from her position in the larger world. In other words, Gilman locates the character narrator in a storyworld in which the rest cure is not an iso-lated medical treatment for her specific post-partum depression but part and parcel of that world's handling of gender and power. Notice here that the consideration of the spatial frame and story space and Gilman's thematizing of them leads into considerations of Gilman's thematizing of the larger storyworld, even though its spatial dimensions are only hinted at. In this connection, also notice that Gilman links one of John's the-matic functions as character with her thematizing of the storyworld. John represents the benevolent patriarch who relies on his gendered authority as husband and as physician to attempt to control his wife's behavior.

Gilman reinforces the relevance of the principle of minimal departure to her story by importing someone from the actual world into her storyworld: Dr. Weir Mitchell, the historical person who prescribed the rest cure to Gilman after she suffered from her own bout of post-partum depression. She has John invoke Mitchell as a threat: "John says if I don't pick up faster he shall send me to Weir Mitchell in the fall" (1396). This line suggests that the character narrator's world is Gilman's world—and by extension the world of her readers in 1892. In this way, the line also calls attention to the significance of the occasion of Gilman's telling. This story matters now because the rest cure is an ongoing abomination.

Three main consequences follow from Gilman's construction of her storyworld as conforming to the actual world:

1   It greatly enhances her efforts to put the mimetic and thematic com-ponents of the space of the house—and the character narrator's experiences of that space—in a feedback loop. That is, this close rela-tionship between the two worlds enables Gilman to make the point that what happens to the character narrator in her storyworld as a result of the rest cure happens to women in the actual world. The more mimetically vivid and arresting Gilman makes the house and the char-acter narrator's experiences of it, the more rhetorical readers will feel the thematic force of both. And the more readers feel that force the more deeply they respond emotionally and ethically to the character narrator's developing experiences.

2   The overlap provides solid ground from which Gilman's rhetorical readers can perceive and judge the character narrator's increasingly dis-torted narration. As noted earlier, if Gilman were to have constructed an alternate rather than a conforming storyworld, she could have opened the door to interpretations in which the character narrator's perceptions and judgments of what is happening behind the wallpaper are signs of her special insights. As it is, though, they are signs of her breakdown, of the way in which the rest cure turns out to be a rest disease.

3   These two points lead to a third about the crucial synthetic function of space in the story. The construction of the character narrator and the construction of the house, the bedroom, and the wallpaper are Gilman's most important building blocks for the story as a whole. Just how much this story depends on the synthetic functions of space becomes clearer when we consider another plausible way for Gilman to construct the story. Rather than making the character narrator's relation to the house its main focus, she could have made the character narrator's relationship with John the main focus—and relegated the house to the background. Gilman's choice, though, brilliantly shows how the character narrator experiences their shared space in ways completely different and entirely unknown to John, even as those experiences are a consequence of his imposing the rest cure on her.

I turn now to develop these three general points through a closer look at their connections to the story's progression and then its bonding unreliability. Gilman signals that space will be a key resource in the opening sentences of the story as the character narrator, speaking in the present tense, remarks how unusual it is for "ordinary people" to rent a "colonial mansion, a hereditary estate," and she wonders whether it is haunted. When she mentions the possibility, she is attracted to the idea: "I would say a haunted house, and reach the height of romantic felicity—but that would be asking too much of fate!" (1392). She then goes on to less happy thoughts and questions:

> Still I will proudly declare that there is something queer about it.
> Else, why should it be let so cheaply? And why have stood so long untenanted?
>
> (1392)

With this opening, Gilman makes the character narrator's relation to the house both an instability and a tension driving the progression. Rhetorical readers move forward interested in (a) how the relation between the character narrator and the house will get complicated and perhaps resolved, and (b) interested in whether Gilman will supply answers to her questions: is the house haunted, either for good or for ill?

Gilman's choice to make the character-space relation central to the progression stands out in relation to other progressions we've seen and to many (most?) others as well. In a great many narratives, the most common kind of global instability is one involving character-character relations. (This generalization applies to the narratives in our group, with the exceptions of "This Old Man" and "One Minus One" because their textual dynamics are governed more by tensions than by the instability—complication—resolution pattern). In such narratives, space has a range of synthetic functions. Authors sometimes use it to complicate those character-character relations as Danticat does with the differences between Carole's and Jeanne's relations to Haiti and the USA in "Sunrise/Sunset." Sometime authors use space to add to the mimetic portraits of their characters: Oates's protagonist reveals much about herself as she imagines transforming her house into a hospice. Authors sometimes use space to add thematic layers to the character-character relations as Tóibín does in "One Minus One" with the geographical distance between the character narrator and Ireland, the home of his former lover. This distance in turn reflects the psychological distance that is itself enacted in the hypothetical nature of the character narrator's phone call. And of course, authors may combine these synthetic functions. Furthermore, when authors do make the protagonist's relation to space a global instability, they typically choose an extraordinary space, such as a wilderness or other unusual landscape, or—wait for it—a haunted house.

Gilman accomplishes a lot with her evocation of the haunted house narrative in her opening. She generates the tension around the possibility that this "hereditary estate" is haunted (is it? if so, why? what's the backstory?—and so on) and ties that tension to the instability (what will be her relation to the house?). Then, by following out the complications of that instability, she resolves the tension in one way for the character narrator and in the opposite way for her rhetorical readers. More specifically, the character narrator believes that the house, though not haunted by a ghost, is hiding a woman behind the yellow wallpaper, and, indeed, perceives greater and greater manifestations of her presence as the story proceeds, until finally her identity merges with that of the woman. By contrast, rhetorical readers, relying in part on the overlap between the storyworld and the actual world and in part on the details of the narration, do not see the house as haunted or the woman behind the wallpaper as real. Instead, they see the character narrator's increasing unreliability about the space as evidence of her psychological unraveling that culminates in her breakdown and loss of identity. Rhetorical readers also recognize that the causes of the character narrator's misperceptions and her breakdown are the rest cure itself and the patriarchal ideology behind it.

Now this summary of the underlying logic of the story's progression is incomplete, and, indeed, I would not be surprised to learn that you think it makes too stark a separation between the character narrator and rhetorical readers. In any case, what's missing is appropriate attention to the readerly dynamics, the trajectory of rhetorical readers' responses to the evolving relationship between the character narrator and the house, the bedroom, and the wallpaper. Crucial to that trajectory is Gilman's use of unreliability, which, I suggest, starts as estranging but becomes increasingly bonding as the character narrator's reporting, interpreting, and evaluating become more egregiously unreliable. Let's take a closer look.

In her initial description of the bedroom, the character narrator, after reliably reporting ("It is a big, airy room") and reasonably interpreting ("it was nursery first and then playground and gymnasium"), she offers this interpretation and evaluation of the wallpaper.

> I never saw a worse paper in my life.
>
> One of those sprawling flamboyant patterns committing every artistic sin.
>
> It is dull enough to confuse the eye in following, pronounced enough to constantly irritate, and provoke study, and when you follow the lame, uncertain curves for a little distance they suddenly commit suicide—plunge off at outrageous angles, destroy themselves in unheard-of contradictions.
>
> The color is repellant, almost revolting; a smouldering, unclean yellow, strangely faded by the slow-turning sunlight.
>
> It is a dull yet lurid orange in some places, a sickly sulphur tint in others.
>
> (1393)

Over and above the particulars, this passage communicates the character narrator's strong negative response to the paper. Gilman marks the narration as unreliable interpreting and evaluating by making the character narrator's complaints incoherent and by having her attribute a strange agency to the paper. It is dull yet irritating; the "lame" curves "commit suicide." Her description of the color(s) is (are) similarly inconsistent: they are "faded" and "dull" yet also "lurid." It is difficult, if not impossible, to construct a clear image of how the paper looks. At this early point in the narrative, the effects of the unreliability are estranging ones, inducing Gilman's rhetorical readers to keep a wary distance from the character narrator's way of viewing her environment.

As the narrative progresses, however, and Gilman reveals more about the rest cure and shows John continually refusing to grant any of the character narrator's requests, including one to change the wallpaper, the effects of the unreliability shift. Gilman establishes the wallpaper as the locus for the character narrator's expression of a feeling that rhetorical readers come to share: something is deeply wrong in this otherwise attractive house. In addition, the increasing unreliability becomes a way for Gilman to trace the transformation of the rest cure into a rest disease and the increasing inability of John to see the character narrator for who she is and to recognize what is happening to her. In all these ways, Gilman affectively and ethically aligns her rhetorical readers with the character narrator and against John.

Gilman deepens these affective and ethical effects by her careful tracing of the character narrator's perception of a woman behind the paper. Consider the following sequence:

> There are things in that paper that nobody knows but me, or ever will.
>
> Behind that outside pattern the dim shapes get clearer every day.
>
> It is always the same shape, only very numerous.
>
> And it is like a woman stooping down and creeping about behind that pattern. I don't like it a bit. I wonder—I begin to think—I wish John would take me away from here!
>
> (1397)

The unreliable interpretation is obvious here, but just as important is her reliably reported response to what she (mis)perceives: she is frightened by the shape that looks like a creeping woman.

A little later, she narrates:

> By moonlight—the moon shines in all night when there is a moon—I wouldn't know it was the same paper.
>
> At night in any kind of light, in twilight, candlelight, lamplight, and worst of all by moonlight, it becomes bars! The outside pattern I mean, and the woman behind it is as plain as can be.
>
> I didn't realize for a long time what the thing was that showed behind,—that dim sub-pattern,—but now I am quite sure it is a woman.
>
> By daylight she is subdued, quiet. I fancy it is the pattern that keeps her so still. It is so puzzling. It keeps me quiet by the hour.
>
> (1399)

Strikingly, now that she clearly identifies the shape as a woman, she is no longer frightened. Gilman invites her rhetorical readers to fill in the gap between the reactions with the inference that she is moving toward an intuitive understanding of something that they have already achieved: the image is not just a woman but a projection of herself. Both are confined, both are restless, yet both monitor their behavior, restricting it at certain times. More than that, it makes psychological sense that the character narrator, so repressed by John, would construct this imaginary double. Indeed, at this point, Gilman is creating bonding effects by inviting her readers to recognize that the character narrator's literal misinterpretation is in many ways metaphorically apt.

Gilman's tracing of the character narrator's perceptions continues:

> I think that woman gets out in the daytime!
>
> And I'll tell you why—privately—I've seen her!
>
> I can see her out of every one of my windows!
>
> It is the same woman, I know, for she is always creeping, and most women do not creep by daylight.
>
> I see her on that long shaded lane, creeping up and down. I see her in those dark grape arbors, creeping all around the garden.
>
> I see her on that long road under the trees, creeping along, and when a carriage comes she hides under the blackberry vines.
>
> I don't blame her a bit. It must be very humiliating to be caught creeping by daylight!
>
> I always lock the door when I creep by daylight. I can't do it at night, for I know John would suspect something at once.
>
> (1400–1401)

Gilman here uses space to show how the character narrator's imaginary double partially acts out her understandable desire for liberation. While the character narrator remains confined to the bedroom and the house, her double can move in the attractive outside spaces she can see from her window. Yet she cannot yet imagine the double's complete liberation: the woman creeps rather than strides, and even more significantly feels compelled to hide herself from the eyes of other people.

The last sentence of the passage is especially poignant because the character narrator begins to merge with her double without realizing it: she becomes the creeping woman. This development shows that the patriarchy warps even the way she acts out her escape at this stage: she must creep and must not be seen creeping. Consequently, as her unreliable interpreting becomes greater, its affective and ethical bonding effects also increase.

Finally, Gilman traces the last step in the character narrator's evolution:

> But here I can creep smoothly on the floor, and my shoulder just fits in that long smooch around the wall, so I cannot lose my way.
>
> Why, there's John at the door!
>
> It is no use, young man, you can't open it!
>
> How he does call and pound!
>
> Now he's crying for an axe.
>
> It would be a shame to break down that beautiful door!
>
> "John dear!" said I in the gentlest voice, "the key is down by the front steps, under a plantain leaf!"
>
> That silenced him for a few moments.
>
> Then he said—very quietly indeed, "Open the door, my darling!"
>
> "I can't," said I. "The key is down by the front door under a plantain leaf!"
>
> And then I said it again, several times, very gently and slowly, and said it so often that he had to go and see, and he got it, of course, and came in. He stopped short by the door.
>
> "What is the matter?" he cried. "For God's sake, what are you doing!"
>
> "I've got out at last," said I, "in spite of you and Jane! And I've pulled off most of the paper, so you can't put me back!"
>
> Now why should that man have fainted? But he did, and right across my path by the wall, so that I had to creep over him every time!
>
> (1402–1403)

This resolution to the progression vividly captures the paradoxes of bonding unreliability. These final steps in the character narrator's merging with her imaginary double indicate that her loss of her own identity is complete. Early in the passage she knows who John is (although perhaps that knowledge flickers when she refers to him as "young man") but by the end she does not. She asks why did "that man" faint rather than asserting something like "John was so upset at the sight of me creeping that he fainted." In this connection, her assertion about getting out "in spite of you and Jane" provides the penultimate step: while she might be referring to John's sister, whom she has previously called "Jennie" and who has been aligned with John, Gilman also allows her audience to interpret "Jane" as the character narrator's name. I favor that interpretation because it fits the pattern of her transformation (and if Gilman wants her readers to think she means "Jennie," why not write "Jennie"?): she continues to be unaware of her merging with the woman from the wallpaper. But the transformation is not yet complete because she can still name John and recognize him as someone trying to contain her.

The last line completes the transformation because she can no longer recognize John: he becomes simply "that man" who fainted, and she does not know why he did. Furthermore, she is affectively indifferent to his fainting, except for the inconvenience it causes her as she creeps around the room. Here Gilman adds another layer to the paradox of bonding unreliability: now that the character narrator has become such an unreliable interpreter and reporter, she is able to shift the power dynamic between herself and John. That shift is reflected first in her having the upper hand in their dialogue and then both literally and symbolically in her crawling over his unconscious body: she dominates this spatial frame. While rhetorical readers welcome this power shift, they retain their sad awareness of its connection to her loss of identity.

More generally, then, in "The Yellow Wallpaper" Gilman generates the progression by making the protagonist's relation to space a global instability, and thus draws on space as a major resource in her construction of the narrative. At the same time, Gilman makes the interaction of space with other resources, especially bonding unreliability, crucial for achieving her affective, ethical, and thematic purposes. It's a remarkably well-crafted and extremely powerful narrative.

Opening Out

Space is an essential resource of narrative because change over time typically also entails change in one or more spaces, and skillful tellers have found—and continue to find—innovative ways to make space function as more than just a background to the action. Furthermore, as we have seen with each of our resources, skillful authors set up productive interactions between space and other resources, and, indeed, sometimes blend space and time in what Bakhtin has called the chronotope. One lesson for caregivers and patients is that the spaces in which their interactions occur are likely to matter and that both therefore should pay attention to them. Patients typically don't have much control over clinics, doctors' offices, and hospitals, and caregivers often don't either. But they can exercise the agency that they do have in ways that put patients' needs and interests first. More than that, caregivers can listen for the functions and influences of space in patients' stories: where things happen—and patients' relations to those spaces—can be as significant as what happens. Thus, for example, in James Rowland's narrative from Chapter 1, caregivers would do well to follow up on his statements that he has experienced chest pains at home and while working out but not at work.

Overstanding Prompt

Respond to this claim: Gilman undermines her critique of patriarchy as manifest in the USA at the end of the nineteenth century by overdoing it. Her character narrator's response to the rest cure is so extreme that Gilman's critique loses its force. Make the case for this position and then respond to it, agreeing or disagreeing, in whole or in part, and giving warrants for your response.

Springboarding Prompts

Rewrite a segment of the story from John's perspective.

Tell a story about a time when you felt that you were in a hostile space.

Tell a story about a time when you were unable to communicate your dissatisfaction—or even distress—to someone who had the power to ameliorate it.

Tell a story about a time when you were in a bad position and were unable to extricate yourself from it.

Tell a story about a time when you were in a bad position and were able to successfully escape to a better one.

Note

1   Ryan, Marie-Laure. "Space." *The Living Handbook of Narratology.*

Works Cited

Bakhtin, M.M. *The Dialogic Imagination*, edited by Michael Holquist, translated by Caryl Emerson and Michael Holquist. Austin, TX: University of Texas Press, 1981.

Gilman, Charlotte Perkins. "The Yellow Wallpaper." In *The Norton Anthology of Literature by Women: The Traditions in English*, 3rd ed., edited by Sandra M. Gilbert and Susan Gubar, 1392–1402. New York: W.W. Norton & Company, 2007 [1892].

Herman, David. *Story Logic: Problems and Possibilities of Narrative*. Lincoln, NE: University of Nebraska Press, 2002.

Oates, Joyce Carol. "Hospice/Honeymoon." *The New Yorker*, 30 July 2020. www.new yorker.com/books/flash-fiction/hospice-honeymoon (Accessed 10 February 2020.)

Ryan, Marie-Laure. "Space." *The Living Handbook of Narratology*, 22 April 2014. www.lhn.uni-hamburg.de/node/55.html (Accessed 11 February 2022.)

Ryan, Marie-Laure, Kenneth Foote, and Maoz Azaryahu. *Narrating Space/Spatializing Narrative: Where Narrative Theory and Geography Meet.* Columbus, OH: Ohio State University Press, 2016.

Stanzel, Franz K. *A Theory of Narrative*, translated by Charlotte Goedsche. Cambridge: Cambridge University Press, 1979.

9 From Print to Comics

Toward a Rhetoric of Graphic Medicine

Graphic narratives about medical issues have become increasingly abundant as graphic narrative itself has become a more widely circulated form. This increasing abundance has given rise to the study of such narratives in the "Graphic Medicine" movement dedicated to the "intersection between the medium of comics and the discourse of healthcare."[1] As with work in narrative theory on space, this movement has emerged from an interaction between narrative practice and narrative theory. The production of comics (following Ian Williams and others, I'll use this term to refer to the medium in which graphic narratives are composed) has a long history, dating back to the rise of newspapers in the nineteenth century and being used for a wide variety of purposes from political satire to light entertainment to serious storytelling (see Gardner). Over the last half-century, comic artists have made both fictional and nonfictional long-form graphic narratives about medical and non-medical subjects an increasingly important use of the medium. An especially notable event was Art Spiegelman's 1980 publication of *Maus*, his innovative and highly praised graphic representation of his father Vladek's experiences in Auschwitz (the title comes from Spiegelman's decision to depict the Jews as mice with the Nazis as cats). Spiegelman's success brought new attention not only to the Holocaust, Holocaust survivors, and their children but also to comics and graphic narrative.

Multiple developments over the last half-century testify to the growing cultural significance of long-form graphic narrative that has in turn contributed to the Graphic Medicine movement. Here is a partial list:

1   As mentioned above, numerous comic artists, including many initially attracted by the medium's status as a subversive form, have produced compelling narratives.
2   Artists and scholars have effectively put to rest the idea that comics are an inferior medium and even one whose corrupting influences make them dangerous reading material for children and teens. Scholars have replaced this idea with the wisdom that skillful artists use the medium to compose narratives that can be as sophisticated, challenging, and rewarding as those rendered in print.

DOI: 10.4324/9781003018865-9

3   Following upon this revisionary view of the medium, scholars have produced a substantial body of work devoted to the theory and interpretation of graphic narrative.

In this chapter, I sketch how the rhetorical prescription for Narrative Medicine I've been writing can be extended to graphic narratives about medical issues by reflecting on the affordances of the comics medium. By affordances I mean the features of the medium that lend themselves to particular kinds of representations and their corresponding effects. In the case of comics these features arise from its visual and verbal tracks of communication and their intertwining. This attention to affordances will lead me to discuss how the medium affects the mimetic, thematic, and synthetic components of narrative as well as the resources discussed in the previous chapters. For reasons of efficiency and clarity, I will discuss them in a different sequence and in four groups: (a) character and progression; (b) space; (c) time; and (d) tellers, perspective, and voice. In each case, everything we've already discussed about these resources remains relevant, but I will emphasize the ways in which the affordances of comics lead artists to use the resources in ways that traditional print does not.

Throughout the discussion, I will consistently refer to two nonfiction graphic memoirs about end-of-life situations. The first is Roz Chast's *Can't We Talk about Something More Pleasant?* in which Chast tells the story of her relationship with her parents, Elizabeth and George, as they cope (and sometimes fail to cope) with multiple challenges during their last years. The second is Miriam Engelberg's *Cancer Made Me a Shallower Person*, in which Engelberg tells the story of her responses to her diagnosis and treatment for breast cancer and of the cancer's eventual metastasis that takes her to the point of death. Chast's and Engelberg's shared commitment to humor helps set in relief many other differences in their handling of the affordances of their medium.

The differences between the narratives are also evident in their progressions and purposes. Chast offers a retrospective and largely chronological account of the last years of her parents' lives (though the narrative is not without analepses and prolepses) a few years after their deaths. Chast has several purposes, some mimetic and some thematic. She wants to give her rhetorical readers a thick description of her experience of her parents' last years so that those readers have a narrative to compare their own experiences with. The occasion and some of the narrating-I's reflections at the time of the telling indicate that she also wants to work through that experience for herself both to better process it and to pay homage to her parents in an honest, non-sentimental way. Chast's ability to achieve her purposes depends on the texture of the narrative itself—panel by panel, page by page—and we'll look more closely at that texture below.

Engelberg's story is a lyric narrative hybrid, though one in which the narrative is the dominant mode. She tells a story of change over time, as it takes her from the onset of her illness to just before her death. In addition, Engelberg clearly marks the main events of the trajectory: diagnosis, surgery, chemotherapy, breast radiation, metastasis, and brain radiation. But Engelberg tells the story not on a single occasion in which she looks back at her overall experience but rather from multiple temporal positions as that experience unfolds. In other words, she tells her story in distinct installments, and sometimes the specific occasion of each installment matters a great deal, as it does when she tells about her initial diagnosis, about her metastasis, and about her final struggle to achieve perspective on her experience (I will look closely at her final struggle later in this chapter). Furthermore, sometimes the installments are miniature narratives; sometimes they are lyric explorations of aspects of her experience; and sometimes they are miniature lyric narrative hybrids.[2] The lyric narrative hybridity of the memoir is crucial to Engelberg's multiple purposes. First, she wants to explore and communicate to her audience multiple dimensions of what's it like to be a cancer patient in the United States in the early twenty-first century. Second, she wants to use both the lyric and the narrative dimensions of the storytelling for therapeutic purposes; she marshals both dimensions in the service of helping her come to terms with her experiences as they unfold while simultaneously offering some comfort to others. Her implicit message is that "I hope sharing my experience, and my ironic take on it, can provide some solace to me and be helpful for others. I especially want to resist the cultural narrative that cancer makes—or should make—one a better person."

Since rhetorical theory defines narrative in general as somebody telling somebody else on some occasion and for some purpose(s) that something happened, it defines the more specific genre of graphic narrative as somebody using the affordances of comics on some occasion and for some purposes to tell somebody else that something happened. What, then, are the affordances of comics?

Scott McCloud, in his influential book, *Understanding Comics*, provides a good starting point with his definition of the medium: "juxtaposed pictorial and other images in deliberate sequence, intended to convey information and/or to produce an aesthetic response in the viewer" (9). As with definitions of narrative, I don't think it's either necessary or wise to seek an ideal definition of comics; instead, I find it more productive to attend to how a definition orients its user to the object defined.[3] In McCloud's case, the orientation is toward particular affordances of the medium: images, juxtaposition, deliberate sequence, and goals. Let's look at his orientation through our rhetorical lenses.

"Juxtaposed pictorial and other images" is McCloud's way of addressing the common characterization of the main affordance of comics: its intertwining of images and text, or, from a rhetorical perspective, its visual and verbal tracks of communication. McCloud's formulation is more fine-grained in two ways: (a) it acknowledges that the verbal track is typically itself a set of images because the graphic artist draws the letters and words composing the text; and (b) it recognizes that comics can have images without text, but not vice versa (though again some panels or pages can be completely given over to narration through drawn letters and words). Reading graphic narrative rhetorically then involves analyzing the effects that arise from the intertwining of the verbal and visual tracks. Or in more formal terms, reading graphic narrative rhetorically involves attending to how the artist on the occasion of their telling handles the interactions of the two tracks in order to accomplish some purposes in relation to an audience. Furthermore, following the a posteriori principle, reading rhetorically means being open to the wide array of relationships between the two tracks: they may reinforce, complement, or contradict each other; they may even, on the surface at the least, seem to be wholly independent of each other.

Reading McCloud's "juxtaposed pictorial and other images" through rhetorical lenses highlights the double meaning of "juxtaposed": images may be juxtaposed *within* a panel and *across* panels. This second meaning highlights the salience of segmentivity as a resource for graphic narrative, and the different ways in which graphic artists can productively use it. Comics typically makes three kinds of page-level segments especially salient:[4] the panel, an image or image(s) plus text typically placed within a bordered frame; the tier, a single row of panels; and the page, the container for the tier or tiers. The page may also be a container for a single panel, called a splash page; or for part of a panel that continues across multiple pages, a spread page. Artists can use the segmentation of storytelling into panels, tiers, and pages to keep rhetorical readers focused on the forward motion of the narrative. But artists can also use segmentation to impede such forward movement and even create some tension in readers between their interests in lingering over individual segments and their interests in the ongoing movement of the narrative. You might think of this tension as the medium prompting you to ask, "should I stay, or should I go?" Furthermore, artists use the visual track to set up additional interactions between the sequence of panels and the overall composition of a page. In other words, the medium encourages attention to both the horizontal flow of communication across tiers and the vertical or "tabular" arrangement of those tiers in the larger unit of the page.[5]

Thierry Groensteen in his *System of Comics* highlights another important layer of comics construction by distinguishing between the artist's uses of breakdown and of braiding. Breakdown refers to the connections and oppositions artists build into juxtaposed panels, and braiding to connections and oppositions they build into non-juxtaposed panels, including ones that may be separated by many pages. Braiding depends on some kind of repetition or echo across panels.

Returning to McCloud's definition, I find that his phrase "Deliberate sequence" highlights his interest not in the single panel cartoon (e.g., Gary Larson's *The Far Side*) but rather in the non-random arrangement of panels.

This orientation influences McCloud's subsequent emphasis on the affordance of the gutter, that is, the space between panels, and the ways it invites audiences to infer temporal, causal, and other kinds of connections between them. Attending to the gutter then is part and parcel of attending to segmentivity at the level of panels and, by extension, to segmentivity at the level of tiers and pages (how many gutters in a tier and on a page). Reading rhetorically also means attending to the effects of an artist's handling of gutters and segments on readerly responses and the relation of those effects to the artist's purposes.

With his closing identification of two broad goals, McCloud moves away from identifying affordances and toward an answer to the so-what question. The breadth of those goals—conveying information and producing an aesthetic response—is in keeping with McCloud's interest in offering a capacious definition of the medium. Each category allows for a wide range of options, that is, all kinds of information and all kinds of aesthetic responses. McCloud's orientation is clearly consistent with rhetorical theory's emphasis on purposes, though rhetorical theory sees purposes as having more layers than McCloud seems to: not just informational or aesthetic but possibly both—and sometimes cognitive, ethical, affective, and others as well.

Mimetic, Thematic, and Synthetic

Comics, more than print, consistently calls attention to its synthetic component. As Jared Gardner points out, one big difference between print and comics is the way each treats the hand of its maker. Print makes that hand and its activity invisible (I'm willing to wager than you haven't once thought about my hands at my keyboard), while comics contains reminders of the artist's hand and their work of constructing the text in every panel. Gardner puts it this way:

> Graphic narrative … does not offer the possibility of ever forgetting the medium, losing sight of the material text or the physical labor of its production. In addition to the artist's line within the figurative representation, we have of course other lines equally fundamental to the comic form: the frame, the gutter, the line around dialogue and thought balloons, the lines of the lettering. Comics is a medium that calls attention with every line to its own boundaries, frames, and limitations—and to the labor involved in both accommodating and challenging those limitations.
>
> ("Storylines," 65)

In other words, the panel, unlike the word, always conveys the message that it is a constructed thing. This conclusion suggests a productive affinity between comics and rhetorical theory: the medium's foregrounding of its construction invites questions about the constructor and their purposes.

This conclusion about the consistent presence of the synthetic, however, does not mean that all graphic narratives always make the synthetic component the most prominent one. Some do, of course. Matt Madden's *99 Ways to Tell a Story: Exercises in Style* is a striking case in point. Madden uses the same raw materials of character, event, time, and space and shapes them into 99 different narratives. (Here's the sequence of events: a man gets up from his computer and walks to his refrigerator; on the way his partner calls down from an upstairs studio, "what time is it?"; he answers, "1:15" and proceeds to the refrigerator. But when he opens the door, he can't remember what he wanted to get from it.) As Madden's title suggests, his exercises with these raw materials subordinate his audience's attention to any one story to his act of constructing 99 versions of it. In a sense, Madden's project is to demonstrate the myriad ways an artist can take advantage of the affordances of comics. But many other graphic narratives make the mimetic and thematic at least as prominent as the synthetic. My accounts of the progression and purposes of Chast's *Can't We Talk* and Engelberg's *Cancer Made Me Shallower* indicate that I regard them as members of this group.

Still, the medium's consistent foregrounding of the synthetic has several significant consequences for mimetic—thematic—synthetic relationships:

1   The synthetic component of character will typically affect the mimetic component in a recognizable manner. The clear evidence of construction serves as a constant reminder that the character is a representation of a person. The same logic applies to representations of objects, spaces, and scenes.

2   At the same time, artists will typically establish a baseline visual style for their representations that also establishes a baseline for their mimetic communications. Thus, for example, Chast's moderate caricature becomes the mimetic norm for her memoir. Establishing a mimetic baseline in turn generates rhetorical readers' affective and ethical engagements with the characters and events of the narrative in a way similar to those engagements in realistic print narrative. Just as in print narrative, these engagements are crucially important for the mimetic-thematic feedback loop. The larger point is that in graphic narrative the mimetic, thematic, and synthetic components are typically all prominent.

3   Furthermore, the specific style of representation typically has some thematic significance. In Engelberg's case, her simple visual style implicitly carries the thematic point that "I'm an ordinary woman." In Chast's case, her style of caricature that generates some of her humor thematizes the need to see the humor in her and her parents' difficult experiences.

4   Artists can take advantage of the consistent attention to the synthetic by easily giving it more prominence than the mimetic or the thematic in any one panel, tier, or page. To put this point another way, in the large class of graphic narratives that make all three components prominent,

rhetorical readers will readily accept the temporary ascendancy of the synthetic over the mimetic and the thematic. For example, Chast deviates from her standard way of representing her mother, Elizabeth, with a panel depicting a "Blast from Chast" in which Elizabeth's head is larger than the bodies of George and Roz (see Figure 10.7 in the next chapter). Chast leaves her baseline mimetic mode for this synthetic one and calls even more attention to herself as the constructor. This feature of the synthetic component in comics lends itself to uses of local fictionality in graphic nonfiction. I'll develop this point in the next chapter.

5   In graphic memoir, the prominence of the synthetic works against the conflation of the author/artist, the narrating-I, and the experiencing-I that often accompanies commentary on print memoir. (In graphic fiction, the temptation to conflate these figures is not as strong as it is in graphic memoir, but, depending on similarities between the artist's and the protagonist's experiences, the temptation can still be present.) In graphic memoir, the experiencing-I is explicitly marked as the artist's constructed and stylized version of their former self. The narrating-I is then that constructed self in the role of retrospective teller. The artist is the agent who constructs both the narrating-I and the experiencing-I.

Character and Progression

I start with these resources because my discussion of them will provide a useful context for my discussion of the other resources. In keeping with the previous section, I focus first on the way comics consistently makes the synthetic component of character prominent.

Chast highlights the synthetic component of her characters in several ways: as noted, she uses a baseline visual style of moderate caricature; she establishes a typical way of drawing each character and then deviates from that standard at different points; and she occasionally juxtaposes her drawings with photographs (more on this strategy of juxtaposition below). Nevertheless, because so many other elements of her narrative ground the characters and events in the actual world and because she represents herself and her parents as having plausible psychological traits, the synthetic and the mimetic comfortably co-exist. Chast uses the synthetic component of her characters to enhance her humor and to highlight various thematic points about the challenges of end-of-life decision-making. More generally, Chast uses the synthetic component of her characters to establish a salutary distance between herself at the time of the telling and her parents and herself at the time of the action. This distance enables her to see Roz, her former self, and her parents with more clarity and humor than Roz was often able to do in the moment.

In addition to her stylized drawings of her parents (see Figures 9.1 and 9.2), Chast goes to great lengths to give full mimetic portraits of each.

My mother was a different story. She was a perfectionist
who saw things in black and white. Where my father was
tentative and gentle, she was critical and uncompromising.

She had once wanted to be a concert pianist, but she said,
"It came too easily to me." She still played at home for
an hour or so every night while my father and I would
cower in admiration on the couch.

She had been an assistant principal in an elementary school
for most of her working life, a job for which she was
perfectly suited. She was good at telling people what to do.
She was decisive, good in a crisis, and not afraid of making
enemies. Those stupid enough to get her angry got what she
liked to call "a blast from Chast."

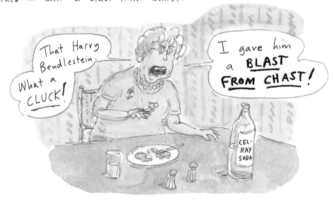

Figure 9.1 Mimetic portrait of Elizabeth

Elizabeth is a formidable person and personality, set in her ways and used to
dominating her husband George, even as she is deeply attached to him.
Elizabeth never established a close relationship with Roz, who throughout
her life feels "far outside [her] parents' duo" (228). George is also set in his
ways and equally attached to Elizabeth, but he is a much kinder and gentler
soul. He does not chafe under Elizabeth's rule, but he is also anxious about
many things. Roz sees her father as "a kindred spirit," but she is also clear-
eyed about George's deficiencies and about both the necessity and difficulty
of supporting her parents as they move through the last years of their lives.
Roz takes on, with varying degrees of reluctance and guilt, the responsi-
bility of seeing them through this period. Roz has complicated feelings
about both her parents, especially her mother, but one of those feelings is
love.

And, more important, he was kind and sensitive. He knew that my mother had a terrible temper, and that she could be overpowering. She had a thick skin. He, like me, did not. She often accused my father of "walking around with his feelers out."

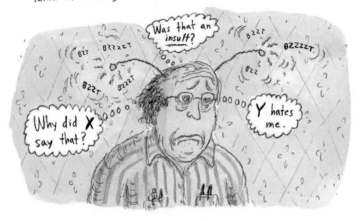

In many ways, my father and I were more alike than my mother and I. We were both only children, and less used to the constant emotional tumult between people than my mother, who was one of five. Also, we were both dilly-dalliers and easily distracted by, say, an interesting word, thereby missing the larger point of what was being said. He often kept me company when my mother was doing other stuff. We watched Twilight Zone together. I'm sure he thought it was dopey, but he knew I loved it, and that I was too scared to watch it alone.

Figure 9.2 Mimetic portrait of George

Engelberg's former self, Miriam, dominates *Cancer Made Me a Shallower Person*. Where Chast's narrative has three protagonists, Engelberg's has just one. Her memoir is all about Miriam's experiences and how the narrating-I processes them. Engelberg highlights the synthetic dimension of Miriam (and her other characters) primarily through the simplicity of her visual style: her drawings pare down actual people to a few salient features. Miriam is primarily drawn with curly hair and glasses on an oval face (see Figure 9.3). Engelberg's visual style encourages her audience to focus on variations within it and on matters of page layout. These variations and layouts interact in multiple ways with the verbal track, and the interactions generate artful ironies about Miriam's experiences that contribute significantly to the mimetic component of her character. Engelberg the artist, Miriam the narrating-I, and Miriam the experiencing-I share a capacity for irony, including self-deprecating irony. While this trait is the most salient

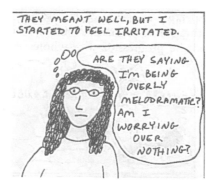

Figure 9.3 Visual image of Miriam

aspect of her mimetic component, its presence along with other aspects of her mimetic situation—as the narrative begins, she is a 43-year-old woman with a husband and a young son, putting together a satisfying life in San Francisco—makes the trajectory of her narrative all the more poignant.

Turning to progression, I note first that if we focus solely on the verbal track and on textual dynamics, then we can carry over the insights from Chapter 3: the verbal track can introduce instabilities and tensions, represent complications, and depict resolutions; it can also play with voice, perspective, temporality, and descriptions of space just as print narratives do. When we expand our focus to include the visual track and especially the interactions of the visual and verbal tracks, we can recognize that skillful artists can take advantage of the affordances of comics to handle textual dynamics—and the synthesis of textual and readerly dynamics—in some additional ways. To take a simple example, once the graphic artist has established their baseline visual style and a default pattern for representing characters, objects, recurrent situations, etc., they can then depart from that default pattern in ways that alter both textual and readerly dynamics. Similarly, artists can establish a standard set of relationships between the verbal and visual tracks (alignment, misalignment, complementarity, etc.) and then can deviate from the standard in order to highlight a particular moment in the textual dynamics. More generally, the multiple options for constructing the interactions between the two tracks give artists a lot of room for creativity.

No small selection of examples can capture the wide variety of ways graphic artists have exercised their creativity. But Chast and Engelberg offer an illuminating sample. With Chast, I will focus on her handling of three different kinds of visual images and their interactions with the verbal track. In the beginning and in the first part of her ending, she juxtaposes photographs and comics (and verbal narration); in the second part of her ending, she adds sketches with minimal verbal narration. With Engelberg, I will focus on her use of the visual track and the gutter to do something remarkable with perspective and temporality in her final installment. In both cases, the resulting textual dynamics have profound effects on the readerly dynamics and the progression as a whole.

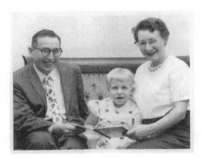

Figure 9.4 The happy Chast family

On p. 2 of *Can't We Talk*, right after her Table of Contents (itself illustrated with her drawings of her parents in their old age), Chast inserts a family photograph (see Figure 9.4). It is a conventional mid-twentieth century photo: a black-and-white image of her father George and her mother Elizabeth in healthy middle-age and Chast herself, sitting between them, at about age five. George and Elizabeth are holding a book open across their daughter's lap and all three are looking up at the camera and smiling. The photograph conveys an image of a unified happy family. Because it follows the Table of Contents, which includes drawings of Roz's elderly parents, the photograph also functions as an analepsis. The significance of the analepsis becomes apparent only as a result of the juxtaposition with the scene depicted in comics on the facing p. 3 (see Figure 9.5).

On that page, Chast initiates her readers into her narratorial dynamics. The baseline visual style of moderate caricature orients her audience to expect a humorous tone. She then relies on the intertwining of the verbal and visual tracks to deliver a funny family scene. But layered beneath that humor are more serious and affectively troubling communications. At this point, Chast uses the visual track to emphasize that her three characters should be thought of less as a group and more as two plus one: Elizabeth and George are always sitting together at one end of the couch while Roz sits at the other end. Furthermore, Chast's repetition of the same basic arrangement of the characters in all eight panels on the page almost makes it into a single large tableau of one (Roz) against two (Elizabeth and George). The funny scene introduces the global instability, which Chast has already pointed to with her title. Chast humorously depicts Roz repeatedly but unsuccessfully trying to get her parents to talk about their plans in case "something **happened**" (part of the humor is that Roz herself speaks only in vague terms). The final panel, split diagonally, with Roz in one half and her parents in the other, shows all three of them expressing their relief about having avoided the difficult conversation by uttering the same word, "Whew!"

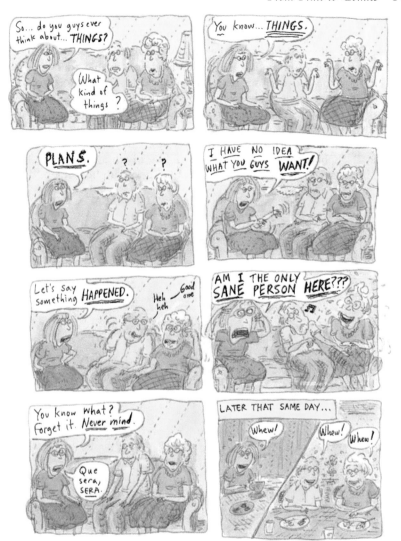

Figure 9.5 Something (not) to talk about

Chast's juxtaposition of the photograph and the comics highlights the synthetic component of her characters and of the narrative as a whole. It also adds to the serious undertone of the humor. First, the photograph grounds the narrative in the world of nonfiction: these moderately caricatured characters are representations of real people. Second, Chast uses the analepsis of the photograph to contrast the past and the present: they were once a unified and happy family (or could at least appear so), but now their threesome has split apart. In addition, they have gone from a stable situation to an alarmingly unstable one: Elizabeth and George are in deep denial about their aging, something Roz recognizes but is, at this juncture, unable to do anything about. And as the last panel suggests, part of her doesn't want to do anything about it. Different kinds of trouble lay in store for all of them.

From p. 3 on, Chast's dominant depiction of Elizabeth is by means of the moderate caricature, though Chast introduces significant variations to help convey the emotions Elizabeth expresses. But at the end of Chapter 17 (p. 202), "Chrysalis" (a term that Chast glosses with a quote from Proust, "death, the chrysalis stage of life"), Chast inserts another photograph, this one

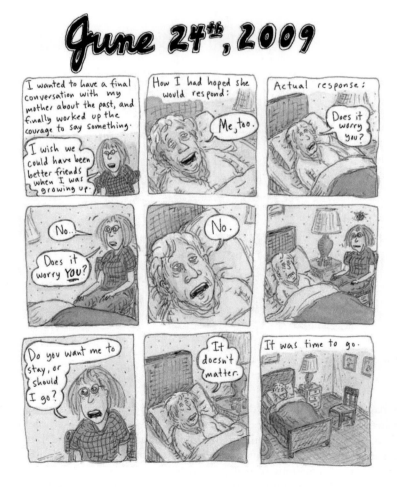

Figure 9.6 A final attempt

of just Elizabeth and Roz, taken when they were only slightly older than they are in the photo on p. 2. Together the photos are an example of how Chast uses braiding to contribute to the progression, since the second one calls back and complicates the first.[6] This second photo follows a page of panels, under the temporal heading of "June 24, 2009," depicting Roz's efforts to have a final heart-to-heart conversation with Elizabeth (Figure 9.6). Roz begins by telling her that "I wish we could have been better friends when I was growing up." When Elizabeth responds not with "me too" but with "does it worry you?" Roz loses her nerve, says no, and the opportunity vanishes. On this page, all but one of the panels shows either Roz or Elizabeth, an indication of their lack of connection. In the only panel depicting both of them, Chast eschews a verbal track as she juxtaposes a distraught Roz with a placid Elizabeth. In the verbal track on the next page, the narrating-I reports that Roz went to her car and cried with a depth of sadness that surprised her.

In the photo, Elizabeth and Roz are about the same age as in the first photo. This one functions as a kind of further revelation of what the family was like when she was a child by focusing on her relationship with her mother. It reveals what the first photo hides. Roz and Elizabeth both look at the camera, but Roz's body is turned toward her mother, as she places her arms around Elizabeth's shoulders in a gentle hug. Elizabeth, however, does not hug her back, but sits placidly looking straight ahead, almost as if Roz isn't there. The photo functions as a sudden analepsis, a reaching back into the past—as if to the time when Elizabeth could have/should have gotten to know her daughter. But the photo suggests that even then it was too late. In so doing, Chast invites rhetorical readers to interpret the scene they've just read as the logical outcome of the scene in the photo: Elizabeth has always already kept Roz at an emotional distance. Chast uses this juxtaposition of scene and photograph as a major part of the resolution in the plot dynamics.

The analepsis of the photograph does not contribute to the plot dynamics (they would be unaffected if Chast did not include it) but it is part of the narratorial dynamics that significantly contributes to the readerly dynamics. The photograph reminds rhetorical readers not only of how much older these real people now are, but also of how little has changed for the better, despite all the time Roz has spent with Elizabeth in these last years of her life. Empathic rhetorical readers may find themselves starting to cry.

Shortly after Chapter 17, however, Chast introduces her third way of depicting Elizabeth and, in so doing, exerts a new influence on the readerly dynamics. Chast includes sketches of Elizabeth that Roz made while keeping vigil near Elizabeth's death bed. Chast's visual style is markedly different in these 13 sketches, with 11 of them getting their own page: the caricature disappears as Roz devotes herself to a more realistic depiction based in her ability to play with light and shadow. As is evident in Figure 9.7, the sketches are also sharply different from the photographs not only because they are marked by the presence of Roz's drawing hand but also because they are

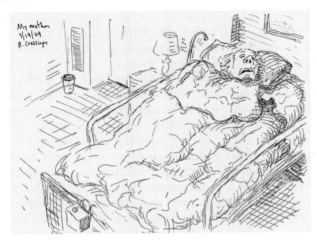

Figure 9.7 Elizabeth in her final days

part of the temporal unfolding of events in the narrative present. In these sketches, Elizabeth lies in bed, her hair has receded, her mouth is in a perpetual frown, and her eyes are closed. The sketches are affectively powerful as they give Elizabeth a kind of dignity in dying that the caricatures would not be able to achieve. More than that, they convey Chast's respect and love for her mother, despite Elizabeth's serious flaws and Roz's regrets about their relationship. In these ways, the sketches add new layers to both the plot dynamics and readerly dynamics because they represent the final events in ways that do not erase Roz's sadness and anger in Chapter 17 but add new feelings to them. These additions in turn deepen rhetorical readers' ethical and affective responses to both Elizabeth and Roz.

Turning to Engelberg, I note that in choosing the strategy of constructing her narrative in installments as her disease advances, Engelberg also faces a considerable challenge in bringing the narrative to a satisfactory ending. She obviously can't narrate her actual death, but ending without any move toward resolution would suggest the narrative was simply cut off. In the installments after her metastasis and in her final one-page installment, "In Perspective" (Figure 9.8), Engelberg handles the challenge in a remarkably effective way.

With the installments after the metastasis, she signals her awareness that she is nearing death in various ways, thus giving greater weight to the occasions of each. First, the effects of the illness become evident in the reduced length of the installments; it's as if she can summon only enough strength to do a page or two at a time. Of her last nine installments, six are only one page, two are two pages, and one is three pages. Yet Engelberg maintains her ability to find irony in her situation. For example, in the penultimate installment, "Bitterness and Envy," Engelberg both admits that

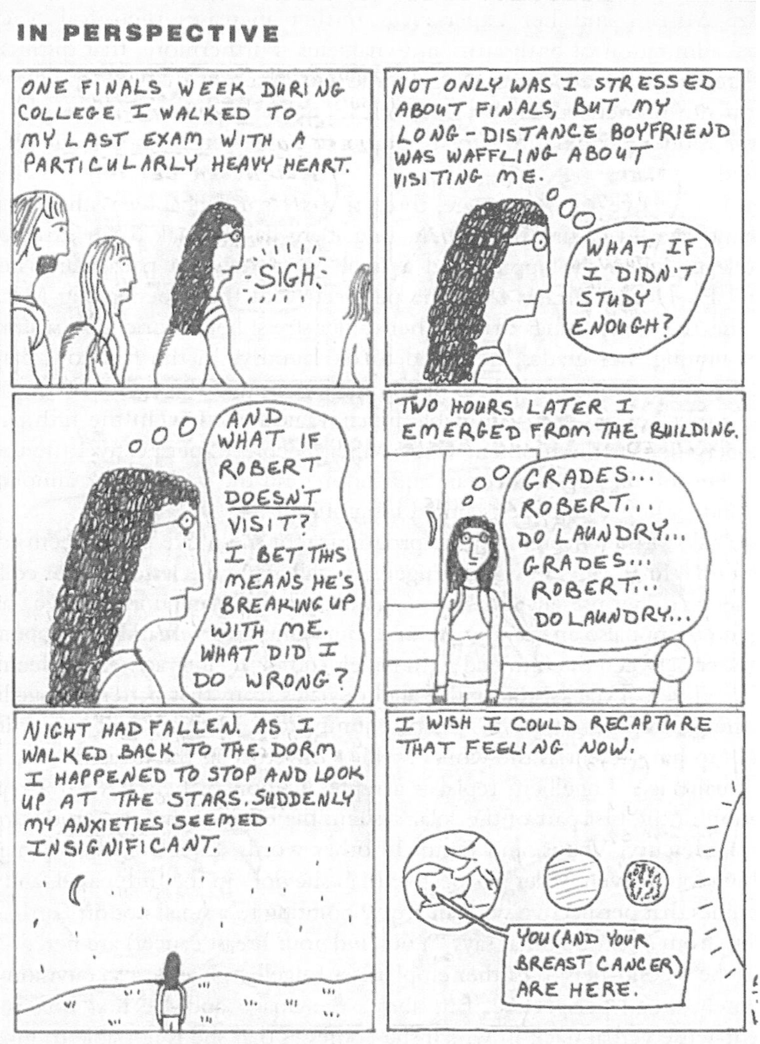

IN PERSPECTIVE

Figure 9.8 Cancer in perspective

she frequently has these feelings and then finds a way to poke fun at herself for having them. Along the way, she also reveals her knowledge of her impending death as she ruminates about things "I'll never get to do."

These chapters deepen the affective and ethical dimensions of the readerly dynamics. Watching Engelberg the artist depict the end stages of life for the Miriam that rhetorical readers have come to admire and feel genuine affection for is itself a wrenching experience. Watching Engelberg continue to

ironize Miriam and her experiences further increases rhetorical readers'
ethical admiration of both artist and character. Furthermore, that distinction
itself begins to break down. Engelberg's construction of these installments
sets up the mimetic-thematic feedback loop: the ordinary Miriam and her
creator model an extraordinary response to Engelberg's knowledge of her
impending death.

"In Perspective" is a one-page, three-tier, six-panel chapter with all panels
the same size. In its first five panels, Engelberg flashes back to an experience
in college, when she approached a final exam "with a particularly heavy
heart." Engelberg narrates from the perspective of the experiencing-Miriam,
who lists the many things that put her under stress: her boyfriend's "waffling"
about visiting, her grades, her need to do laundry. In the first four panels,
Engelberg uses Miriam's lack of discrimination among the causes of her stress
to construct her less-than-admirable psychological portrait. In the fifth panel,
Engelberg depicts the moment when Miriam achieves perspective: the image
shows her looking up at the stars and moon, and the verbal track announces
that "suddenly my anxieties seemed insignificant."

The title of the chapter and the progression of these five panels seem to be
setting up a final panel in which Engelberg will apply the lesson of her college
experience to her present situation. A familiar rather than an innovative narrative pattern, but also an appropriate one. But something remarkable happens in
the gutter between the fifth and sixth panels and in the interaction between the
visual and verbal tracks: the sixth panel deviates from that pattern. Engelberg
uses the gutter as a device to abruptly jump from Miriam's past as a college
student to her present as the woman telling this story in the present tense. On
the visual track, Engelberg replaces a representation of herself with a representation of the first part of the solar system: the edge of the sun, crude drawings of Mercury, Venus, and Earth. In other words, Engelberg shows herself
reaching for an even wider perspective than she does in the fifth panel, and she
underlines that perspective with an arrow pointing to a small dot on Earth, and
coming from a text box that says "You (and your breast cancer) are here." The
use of the second-person further emphasizes Engelberg's ability to envision this
extremely broad perspective. But above the image and the text box is the
present-tense verbal track in which she confesses that she is not able to inhabit
that perspective: "I wish I could recapture that feeling now."

This installment is such an effective ending because it implicitly acknowledges the lure of the master narrative that will allow her to claim some kind of
mastery over her situation ("I am suffering but I can put that suffering in a
larger perspective") and then repudiates that master narrative in favor of a more
honest but far less comforting note: my suffering now is so great that I cannot
achieve the kind of perspective that I once had. Although the disparity
between text and image may initially appear to be another stroke of Engelberg's irony, I find that she invites her audience to read beyond that appearance
to the pairing of two non-ironic communications: I'm aware of the perspective
that could help me out, but I'm unable to achieve it. The best I can do is wish

for it. And there's an additional invitation to her rhetorical readers to oscillate between the perspective she strives for and her inability to achieve it.

This lyrical exploration of perspective gets additional force from its position as the last chapter. Engelberg's telling ends on this unfilled wish, which becomes a marker of her final days, and leaves her audience to contemplate both what happens next and the texture and quality of what has already happened.

Represented Space and the Spatial Layout of Pages

As with the other resources, the concepts relevant to space in print narrative are also relevant to its nature and function in comics. The constructs of spatial frame, story space, setting, storyworld, and narrative universe all apply. Thus, for example, in Chast the story space is composed of four main spatial frames: the Brooklyn apartment in which George and Elizabeth have lived since they were married; Maimonides Hospital; the assisted living facility (aka "The Place") to which they move and in which they both die; and Roz's house in Connecticut. The main setting, then, is New York City and suburban Connecticut in the early 2000s. The storyworld is the United States. The narrative universe extends to include the alternative world in which Roz has a happier relationship with her parents, especially her mother.

Along the visual track, however, artists will always offer a perspectival approach to space, since the drawing will always imply a look from somewhere. In *Can't We Talk?* for example, Chast constructs a perspectival map as she draws a snapshot of part of the Brooklyn neighborhood where she spent her unhappy childhood and where her parents still live. She depicts a series of ugly store fronts, from a vantage point across the street, reinforcing their ugliness by giving them names such as "Smelly Old Groceries" and "Grim Dress Shop" (19).

Comparing Chast's narrative with Engelberg's also underlines another point of rhetorical theory's Authors—Resources—Audiences model. Different authors will make some resources more prominent than others, depending on their purposes. While both Chast and Engelberg make spatial layout important, Chast does far more with the intersection between represented space and spatial layout than Engelberg does. While it would be possible to identify the spatial frames of Engelberg's narrative, and while some panels such as "In Perspective" do significant things with the intersection between represented space and the spatial layout of her pages, Engelberg gives far less attention to the spaces in which Miriam's experiences happen than Chast does to the spaces in Roz's life. In the rest of this section, then, I will focus primarily on Chast's use of space.

One of the main affordances of comics is that it sets up interactions between represented space and the material space of the page. To put the point another way, the spatial layout of the page (which includes the handling of space in panels and tiers) is itself a rich resource for artists to use in the service of their communicative purposes. The length and width of the page can vary from one book to the next (another sign of the importance of the macro-structure), but the default within any one book is that all pages are equal, because they all have the same length and width. Consequently, artists can signal the relative importance of any aspect of their narrative (an event, a character's expression, a narrator's reflection, etc.) according to how they use the spatial layout of the page to represent it. The default relation between aspect and layout is that more space—a larger panel, multiple panels devoted to the same aspect—signals greater importance. Splash pages such as Engelberg's chapter "Everything Is My Enemy," which comes before her metastasis and which I'll discuss in detail in the section on Time, are a good example (Figure 9.9). Engelberg uses the splash page itself to declare that she regards this ironic representation of her paranoia

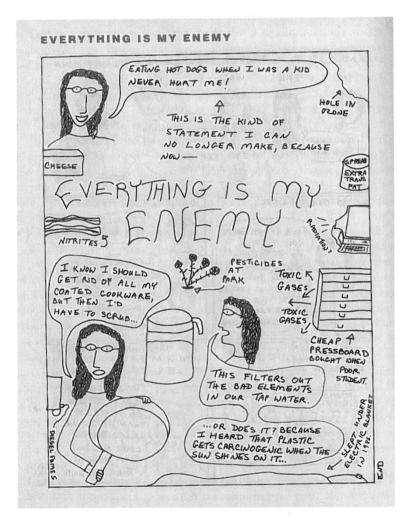

Figure 9.9 Everything is my enemy

as an important part of her story. By making the single page a chapter, she further underlines its importance: the message is that this one-page segment has the same weight in her overall communication as that of any other chapter, including those that are six pages (her longest chapters).

These points, along with previous observations about the page as a whole unit with potentially interacting horizontal and vertical or tabular organization and Groensteen's concept of breakdown (to describe the linear relationships among panels), provide the ground for a closer look at Chast's page from Chapter 17 (Figure 9.6).

The heading, "June 24th, 2009," is in bold script and extends across most of the top of the page. These features, in combination with the fact that this is the first time Chast has used a date as a heading, marks the scene to follow as a momentous one. It's as if the date is seared in her memory.

The rest of the page is divided into three tiers with three panels in each tier, and all nine panels are the same size. I previously noted how Chast uses the linear movement of the panels to emphasize the emotional distance between Elizabeth and Roz, despite their physical proximity. In eight of the nine panels only one of them is present, and, in the exception, they sit in silence. In that panel, Chast emphasizes Roz's feelings of hurt and rejection through her facial expression and the black ball of frustrated feeling above her head.

Attending to the tabular dimension of the page, I notice two significant features:

1   The contrast between the first panel and the last. In the first, Chast gives a close-up image of an eager Roz and uses the verbal track to express the perspectives of both the narrating-I ("I wanted to have a final conversation") and the experiencing-I ("I wish we could have been better friends"). In the last, Roz is absent, and the visual image of Elizabeth lying in her bed is from a more distant perspective and the colors are faded. Chast uses the verbal track for a simple statement by the narrating-I from the perspective of the experiencing-I: "It was time to go." In short, Chast uses the spatial layout to show that Roz's efforts to get closer to her mother end up increasing their emotional distance.

2   Chast uses the three-by-three grid not only to divide the scene into nine equal beats but also to set up three vertical patterns. The column on the left shows three visual images of Roz speaking to her mother; the one in the middle shows three images of Elizabeth responding to Roz; and the one on the right a sequence of Elizabeth responding to Roz, Elizabeth plus Roz sitting in silence, and finally Elizabeth lying by herself underneath the narrating-I's "It was time to go."

In all these ways, Chast uses the intersection of the represented space of Elizabeth's room with the spatial layout to convey the pain and rejection Roz feels in the scene, and to set up the reflections on the verbal track on the next page that I analyzed in the section on progression.

The default of more space on the page signaling more emphasis on what's represented in that space also applies to the proportion of a page, tier, or panel devoted to the verbal track or the visual track. Indeed, artists can make the spatial layout of a page signify even when the page does not contain any visual representation of space. In the last two pages of *Can't We Talk*, Chast restricts herself to the verbal track as she reflects on the events of the memoir and on her relationships with her parents more generally. While Chast has made ample use of the verbal track in the memoir—sometimes even giving more of a page to it than to her visuals—she has only once before restricted herself to that track for as long as two pages: in the chapter "Post-Mortem," immediately following the death of George. She uses those two pages to recount her taking Elizabeth to Roz's house in Connecticut where Elizabeth suffered the indignity of losing control of her bowels. These two unusual instances of giving two pages exclusively to the verbal track invite rhetorical readers to look for braiding effects, despite the overt differences in the content of the verbal track.

Here are the final sentences:

> [My parents] still appear in my dreams. In the ones with my mother, I am usually about to go somewhere with my friends or my husband or my kids, but suddenly, she begins to collapse and I have to take care of her. My father usually appears sitting at our kitchen counter, drinking tea, and reading the newspaper, and he is not worried.
>
> (228)

Chast could have juxtaposed these descriptions with visual images, but by opting not to, she creates two main effects, the first of which follows from the spatial braiding. Just as Chast paused the visual track after the death of George, she now turns away from it for good after the death of Elizabeth. In other words, by not including the images, Chast emphasizes the absence of her parents from her life. They appear to Roz but only in dreams. The second effect follows from the first. By restricting herself to the verbal track, Chast trades the caricature and humor typically accompanying her visuals for the consistently somber tone of her time-of-the-telling voice. This tone and her candid reporting provide an effective ending because they underline the differences in Chast's coming to terms with her relationships with each parent and with the events of their last years. With her mother, the process of coming to terms is ongoing, whereas with her father, she has achieved a kind of peace and acceptance that she indirectly reveals by projecting it onto him: "he is not worried."

Time

Addressing time in comics means attending not just to order, duration, frequency, and the occasional fuzziness of each but also to the gutter and to the segmentivity of tiers and pages.

As McCloud and others point out, a lot happens in the gutter. Or to put this point rhetorically, gutters prompt a lot to happen in the authorial audience's processing of a graphic narrative. McCloud emphasizes how much happens in the gutter by using the term "closure" to describe the reader's filling in the gaps between panels—the gutter opens a space between panels and then the reader closes it with some interpretation. I don't want to adopt McCloud's term because I find "closure" to be more apt for the discussion of narrative endings, but I do endorse his claims about the gutter's prompting of readerly inference.

The most common inference to make about what happens in the gutter is that time passes. This inference follows from the default convention that the progression of panels corresponds to a progression through time: each segment of the narrative unfolding in the panels corresponds to a different moment, and, unless marked otherwise, each moment follows the previous one. Thus, for example, in Engelberg's "In Perspective," the first five panels represent a sequence of events on the day the college-age Miriam took her exam, with each panel detailing a later event than the previous one. But "In Perspective" also demonstrates that the temporal interval between panels can vary widely with little or no explicit calling out of that variation. When Engelberg moves from the fifth to the sixth panels she moves forward approximately 30 years with no other signal than the word "now" in the verbal track (and though the "now" adds clarity, Engelberg could have conveyed the 30-year jump just by shifting from past to present tense in the verbal track).

Furthermore, "In Perspective" also shows that our understanding of temporality in any one installment of *Cancer Made Me Shallower* typically depends on the installment's relation to the rest of the narrative. Because Engelberg has previously established the primary narrative to be the story of her illness and treatment, the first five panels of "In Perspective" constitute an analepsis. Thus, what happens in the gutter between the fifth and sixth panels is not just that 30-year jump but also a return to the primary narrative—and as I've discussed earlier in the section on Character and Progression a return that sets up Engelberg's moving ending.

Chast offers another striking example of the interactions among the gutter and time in a sequence of panels explicitly about time. Among other things, this example shows Chast taking advantages of the affordances of the medium to do something creative with duration. In order to capture what it was like to wait with Elizabeth for treatment in the Emergency Room of Maimonides Hospital, Chast uses a sequence of seven panels, each with a different image of a clock and each framed with verbal commentary either on the passing of time or the hospital environment (Figure 9.10). Furthermore, she spreads the seven panels across the last three of the four three-panel tiers on the page (two in tier two; all of tier three; and two in tier four). This layout both separates this account of what it was like to wait and connects it to the ongoing activity of the hospital.

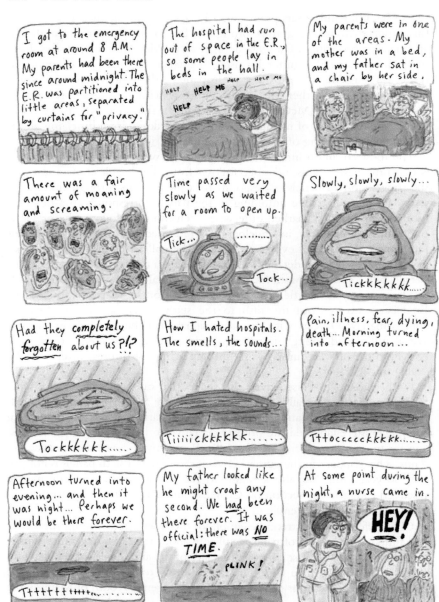

Figure 9.10 Subjective time

In the first panel, the verbal frame is "Time passed very slowly as we waited for a room to open up," and the image is of a clock, drawn with a face (two eyes, a nose that is also the meeting point of the two hands, and a mouth), saying "Tick …" "……." and "Tock … ." The hands of the clock indicate that it is 12:35. In this panel, Chast is playing with the default convention of using one panel to capture one moment in time in order to convey the difference between clock time and subjective time. On the one hand, the clock literally shows a single moment, but on the other, the "……." between "Tick" and "Tock" and the verbal track insist that time is passing for Roz and her parents without it being registered on the clock.

In the next panel, the hands of the clock have moved to 12:40, but the verbal track emphasizes that they move "Slowly, slowly, slowly … ." And the clock, now no longer completely round, says only a long drawn out "Tickkkkkkk." Chast uses the gutter to invite her readers fill in how much subjective time has passed in those five minutes. There's no definitive answer, but rhetorical readers can confidently say "way more than five minutes."

As the sequence continues, Chast further deforms the image of the clock, showing it gradually collapsing on itself until its original circle becomes a line and then disappears altogether. Accompanying this deformation in the clock's shape is a decline in its ability to say "Tick/Tock" until in the sixth panel it says only "Tttttttttttttt…" and, in the seventh, when she declares in the verbal track that "it was official: there was NO TIME," the clock becomes a disappearing dot that makes a final "plink" as it vanishes.

In sum, Chast uses the sequence to dramatize the yawning gap between two kinds of duration: that of clock time and that of her and her parents' subjective experience of time while waiting to be seen. The sequence works so well because Chast's handling of the gutters and segmentivity brings in a third kind of duration: that of the telling. I won't argue that seven segments across three of the four tiers on the page is the perfect number perfectly arranged (if there were six or eight panels and a somewhat different layout, I don't think any of us would contend that Chast should have used seven). Nevertheless, I say with confidence that three or four panels across a single tier would be insufficient and that ten or eleven (with some spilling on to the next page) would be too many. Seven across three tiers allows Chast to drag out the telling so that her rhetorical readers can get a sense of her characters' experience of subjective time without making readers feel as if her representation of that experience is itself interminable. Just as important, by using the gutters to keep the temporal intervals between panels indeterminate, Chast reinforces the point about subjective time. By making it impossible to determine how many hours they waited, she signals that the answer doesn't matter. What matters is that they felt like time eventually disappeared.

In Engelberg's splash page chapter, "Everything Is My Enemy" (Figure 9.9), she offers an example of how to use a single panel to convey multiple moments in time as well as the indeterminate layering of some of those moments to construct a fuzzy temporality. Engelberg fills the page with multiple images, including three of her experiencing-I, along with statements by her inside speech balloons and two present-tense statements from her narrating-self, one of which repeats the title of the installment. This busyness on the page reflects the unsettled feelings conveyed by that title.

More specifically, Miriam says in a speech bubble at the top of the page, "Eating hot dogs when I was a kid never hurt me" and her other two statements are in the form of "I should do X, but Y." Because Engelberg draws her experiencing self the same way in all three images, she invites her rhetorical readers to think that each statement comes from the same temporal location. But just under the speech bubble at the top of the page, Engelberg inserts another present-tense comment: "This is the kind of statement I can no longer make, because now——." That comment destabilizes the temporal location of the opening statement, since both are present tense but the second one seems "more present." Should rhetorical readers now regard the first statement as something Miriam uttered in the past? But what would be her motivation?

Engelberg fills the visual track with a large and not very coherent set of images of inimical objects: hot dogs, a hole in the ozone, cheese, transfat, pesticides in the park, a filter for tap water, an electric blanket, and more. Some of these are part of her current environment, some may or may not be, and some, like the electric blanket, which she describes in the verbal track as something she slept under in 1998, are part of her past. But the title and its repetition in large letters in the middle of the page indicate that she regards all the objects as her enemy *now*. In this way, she layers the past on to the present.

Engelberg marshals her handling of time in the service of her complex ironic communication on this page. Rhetorical readers may initially conclude that she must be straightforwardly ironic, because the set of objects is such an ad hoc collection. Engelberg surely does not want her audience to take her literally about that electric blanket. Nevertheless, a little reflection suggests that, just as surely, she does not want her audience to totally reject her literal meaning. Some of these things—and others not depicted in the list but part of "everything"—are indeed her enemy. Furthermore, her handling of time helps convey the actual paranoia of her experiencing self, and, for that reason, her audience needs to take the literal meaning of the title seriously. At the same time, the irony indicates that Engelberg as author recognizes Miriam's paranoia and can poke fun at it. In other words, the panel shows her remarkable ability to negotiate both the literal and ironic channels of communication as well as her ability to retain some difference between herself as artist and Miriam as experiencing character. In so doing, Engelberg both exposes the limitations of her experiencing self and displays her capacity to step back and ironize that self. This observation leads to another one about Engelberg's telling in time. As she constructs this chapter, Engelberg achieves the kind of perspective that she so poignantly but unsuccessfully strives for later as she constructs "In Perspective."

Tellers, Perspective, and Voice

Again, much of what I've said previously about these resources is relevant to comics even as the affordances of comics lead to some important differences in how they typically get deployed. The somebody telling is the author-artist and, in cases such as the comics of Harvey Pekar whose visual tracks were drawn by R. Crumb, the two flesh-and-blood agents typically collaborate so that they form a single implied author-artist. In other words, while actual readers may be aware of the two agents, from the perspective of the authorial audience, they are a team that functions as a single agent. That author-artist, in turn, constructs a narrating-I who can employ their perspective at the time of the telling or the perspective of a character (experiencing-I or, in fiction, an invented character) at the time of the action. The author-artist also constructs characters whose dialogue at the time of the action contributes to the telling in ways that I've previously discussed. The voices of the narrating-I and of characters will also signify in the ways that they do in print narrative.

But comics complicates these relationships in two main ways:

1   Comics often juxtaposes within a single panel the voices of the narrating-I, via a text box at the top of the panel, and the characters, via speech or thought balloons. Because the voices are contained within a single panel, the artist sets up layered, interactive relationships between them.
2   The layering of voices also interacts with a layering of perspectives. In addition to the layering of *temporal* perspectives that corresponds with the layering of voices, comics always includes an angle of vision along the visual track. This angle may vary along numerous spectra: it may follow a character's gaze; it may be external to the character; it may depict the character looking as well as what the character sees; it may offer views from the side or views from the front; it may be close up or distant; it may be sharp or blurry; and so on. But some visual perspective is inevitable.[7]

Not every panel will juxtapose all these voices and perspectives, but many will. Furthermore, the juxtapositions across panels can also lead to significant interactive effects. The affordances of the medium for the author-artist's deployment of voice and perspective contribute greatly to the medium's semiotic richness.

These general points should become clearer when we analyze how the juxtapositions work on page 201 of *Can't We Talk* (Figure 9.6). I will focus primarily on the heading, the first panel, and the last tier. I invite you to select a page from *Cancer Made Me Shallower* and do a similar analysis (the chapters "Valium in the Workplace," "You Look Good," and "Survivor" are all worth a closer look).

The heading, "June 24, 2009," is in the voice and perspective of the narrating-I, and together with the bold script, signals how the date remains a momentous one for her. At the top of the first panel, Chast uses the voice and perspective of the narrating-I: "I wanted to have a final conversation with my mother about the past, and finally worked up the courage to say something." From the middle to the bottom, she uses the voice and perspective of the experiencing-I: "I wish we could have been better friends when I was growing up." In this way, the narrating-I provides the context for the experiencing-I's appeal to her mother. The angle of vision is on Roz, whose gaze in turn is directed at her mother—as rhetorical readers infer from both the narrating-I's comment and the page as a whole. As for the voices, the narrating-I speaks frankly to her narratee about how difficult this effort was for Roz (think back to the "Whew" of page 3), who takes the risk of talking about something potentially but not necessarily unpleasant. Roz's voice, as she talks to Elizabeth, combines wistfulness with candor. Chast, in short, uses voice and perspective to pack a lot into the panel.

The narrating-I's comment in the first panel functions as a frame for the rest of the scene as it gets played out over the next seven panels and as it depicts Roz's final rejection by Elizabeth. In the third tier, Chast uses the dialogue of Roz and Elizabeth across the first two panels of the tier as a way to capture this culminating moment of Roz's relationship with Elizabeth. Roz asks about Elizabeth's preference, "Do you want me to stay, or should I go?" and Elizabeth responds, "It doesn't matter." The visual perspectives also subtly interact. In the first one, Chast offers an external close-up of Roz (she takes up more space in this panel than in any of the other three in which she appears), even as she continues to show Roz looking at Elizabeth. In the second, Chast offers Roz's angle of vision on Elizabeth, but rather than giving a close-up, she depicts Elizabeth as further away from Roz than ever before. In this way, Chast uses the visual perspective to underline the emotional distance depicted in the dialogue. In the final panel, Chast moves the perspective a little further away from Elizabeth and the now empty chair beside her bed. The angle of vision is no longer Roz's but rather that of the retrospective narrating-I whose voice also returns: "It was time to go." So sad.

Opening Out

As comics in general and graphic medicine in particular continue to receive so much well-deserved and valuable attention from scholars, our understanding of the interaction between the medium and the discourse of health care will continue to grow. Conceiving of graphic narrative as rhetoric will contribute to that growth even as the practices of graphic artists will continue to extend the explanatory power of rhetorical theory. Furthermore, caregivers and patients may want to experiment with communicating via comics. Just as oral storytelling in the clinic need not approach the aesthetic quality of the print narratives we've examined in this book to be effective, comics storytelling need not be as artful as Chast's and Engelberg's to add value to the clinical encounter.

Overstanding Prompts

Respond to the following claim: Chast's ambition to represent her deeply mixed feelings of love, exasperation, guilt, and so on is admirable but not ultimately successful. Underneath the overt story and all its humor is a more revealing one. Her parents did not love her, and she did not love them. Consequently, she acts primarily out of guilt and obligation, and her humor cannot paper over how miserable she and her parents are throughout the story. Make the case for this position and then respond to it, agreeing or disagreeing, in whole or in part, and giving warrants for your response.

Respond to the following claim: Engelberg's self-deprecating irony is a subtle way of boasting about her response to her diagnosis. Her position is not that cancer made her shallower but that it gave her the opportunity to be noticed and praised that she always longed for. Make the case for this position and then respond to it, agreeing or disagreeing, in whole or in part, and giving warrants for your response.

Springboarding Prompts

Try your hand at graphic storytelling by taking a scene from either *Can't We Talk?* or *Cancer Made Me Shallower* and retelling it in your own visual style and with any other changes you'd like to make.

Tell a story—in prose or in comics—about an important conversation you had with one of your parents or with another family member.

Tell a story—in prose or in comics—about receiving bad news and how you responded to it.

Tell a story—in prose or in comics—about something you regret and that you know you can't do anything to change.

Tell a story—in prose or in comics—about a struggle to attain what you regarded as a healthy perspective on some event(s) in your life.

Notes

1 The statement comes from Ian Williams on the Graphic Medicine website www. graphicmedicine.org. This website is now maintained by Graphic Medicine International Collective, a scholarly society founded in 2019 that also hosts an annual conference. Some founding members of the Collective, M.K. Czerwiec, Ian Williams, Susan Merrill Squier, Michael J. Green, Kimberly R. Myers, and Scott T. Smith, co-authored *The Graphic Medicine Manifesto* in 2016.

2 Engelberg frequently uses her chapter titles to signal whether her goals in each are primarily lyric, primarily narrative, or hybrid. "Diagnosis," for example, signals narrative, while "Luck" indicates lyric, and "Waiting" lyric narrative.

3 In this respect, my general position about defining comics is similar to but not identical with the one offered by Kai Mikkonen in *The Narratology of Comic Art*. Mikkonen finds it unnecessary to define comics, since existing definitions,

including McCloud's, can all be regarded as inadequate in some way. He finds it better to state that there is a substantial and recognized corpus of individual works in the mode and not worry about the fine points of stipulating the relation between its visual and verbal components. My position is not identical to Mikkonen's because I make a case for the practical utility of a rhetorical definition.

4 Graphic narrative can and often does also work with larger segments: chapters, parts, the book itself. But in keeping with this book's interest in close reading/attentive listening, I will focus primarily on the more fine-grained uses of segmentivity across panels, tiers, and pages.

5 Jan Baetens and Hugo Frey have an excellent chapter on page layouts in *The Graphic Novel: An Introduction.*

6 More generally, Chast uses seven family photographs to set up a complex braid that invites comparison across the photographs and between each photo and its surrounding context. Chast also uses another set of photographs of the stuff her parents leave behind when they move out of their apartment. This set is better understood as an example of what Groensteen calls breakdown because its effects arise from the linear presentation of all this accumulation.

7 For an excellent deep dive into these matters, see Horstkotte and Pedri.

Works Cited

Baetens, Jan and Hugo Frey. *The Graphic Novel: An Introduction.* New York: Cambridge University Press, 2014.

Chast, Roz. *Can't We Talk about Something More Pleasant?* London: Bloomsbury, 2014.

Czerwiec, M.K., Ian Williams, Susan Merrill Squier, Michael J. Green, Kimberly Myers, and Scott T. Smith. *The Graphic Medicine Manifesto.* University Park, PA: Penn State Press, 2015.

Engelberg, Miriam. *Cancer Made Me a Shallower Person.* New York: Harper Collins, 2006.

Gardner, Jared. *Projections: Comics and the History of Twenty-First Century Storytelling.* Palo Alto, CA: Stanford University Press, 2012.

Gardner, Jared. "Storylines." *SubStance* 40, 1 (2011): 53–69.

Groensteen, Thierry. *The System of Comics.* Jackson, MI: University Press of Mississippi, 2007.

Horstkotte, Silke and Nancy Pedri. *Experiencing Visual Storyworlds: Focalization in Comics.* Columbus, OH: Ohio State University Press, 2022.

Madden, Matt. *99 Ways to Tell a Story: Exercises in Style.* New York: Penguin, 2005.

McCloud, Scott. *Understanding Comics.* New York: Harper Collins, 1994.

Mikkonen, Kai. *The Narratology of Comic Art.* New York: Routledge, 2017.

10 Fictionality

In previous chapters, we have been considering both fictional and nonfictional narratives. (Just to review, the fictional narratives are the two stories by Oates, Selzer's "Imelda," Tóibín's "One Minus One," Danticat's "Sunrise/Sunset," and Gilman's "The Yellow Wallpaper"; the nonfictional stories are Tweedy's "People Like Us," Angell's "This Old Man," Wolff's "Close Calls," Chast's *Can't We Talk about Something More Pleasant?*, and Engelberg's *Cancer Made Me A Shallower Person*.) In Chapter 1, I offered a brief demonstration of the consequences of understanding Oates's "Widow's First Year" as fictional or nonfictional. In this chapter, I take up the question of how authors of both fiction and nonfiction can use the resource of fictionality (departures from the direct representation of actual events—fuller definition to follow) to achieve their purposes with different audiences. I am especially interested in local uses of fictionality by authors of global nonfictions, since they help illuminate the pervasiveness of fictionality and the advantages of taking a rhetorical approach to it. After a brief analysis of Selzer's handling of the character narrator's turn toward fictionality in "Imelda," I will take up Tobias Wolff's use of it in the "Close Calls" chapter of *In Pharaoh's Army* and then Chast's deployment of it in *Can't We Talk?*

On the surface, it seems that the key differences between nonfiction and fiction are ontological: one deals with things that exist, and the other with things that are invented or imagined. Hence, nonfiction is tethered to the actual world, and fiction is not. This way of thinking sets up fiction and nonfiction as binary opposites, different discourses doing different things in relation to different worlds. While acknowledging the viability of the ontological approach for some questions, rhetorical theory takes a more pragmatic approach, one characteristically grounded in attention to purposes. From this pragmatic perspective, both fiction and nonfiction ultimately want to influence the way audiences think, feel, and act in and about the actual world. Consequently, rhetorical theory regards fiction and nonfiction as different means to similar ends. Nonfiction's means are direct, while those of fiction are indirect.[1]

This rhetorical, pragmatic approach leads to the following definitions. Nonfictionality is discourse in which somebody reports, interprets,

DOI: 10.4324/9781003018865-10

evaluates, or otherwise engages with actual states of affairs in order to influence somebody else's understanding, beliefs, attitudes, or feelings about those states of affairs and/or to persuade them to take some action about those states. Fictionality is discourse in which somebody intentionally invents, projects, or otherwise directs somebody else to imagine non-actual states of affairs in order to influence that audience's understanding, beliefs, attitudes, or feelings about actual states of affairs and/or to persuade them to take some action about those states.

Two other important points follow from these definitions. First, from a rhetorical perspective, fictionality is fundamentally different from lying because it is not deceptive. The somebody using fictionality wants the audience to recognize their departure from the actual, while the liar does not. In other words, the liar presents their utterance as an instance of nonfictionality. From this perspective, then, the discovery of a lie does not transform it into an instance of fictionality but exposes it as a deceptive instance of nonfictionality. Second, in addition to fictionality, nonfictionality, and lying, rhetorical theory recognizes discourses that deliberately blur the lines between fictionality and nonfictionality for their own purposes. Autofiction such as J.M. Coetzee's trilogy, *Boyhood, Youth, Summertime* is an excellent example. In such narratives the question of whether a specific event actually happened in just the way it is represented becomes beside the point, since the point is that the representation of the event helps illuminate the writer's life.

This pragmatic approach also opens up the difference between fictionality and nonfictionality as modes of discourse, and fiction and nonfiction as macro-genres of narrative. In other words, fictionality is not confined to generic fiction but is pervasive in discourse. Once you start looking for it, you can't miss it. It's in television commercials that make inanimate things animate (the Geico gecko!), in political campaign speeches that predict a rosy future (Build Back Better!), in philosophical thought experiments that highlight ethical dilemmas (the Trolley Problem!), and in doctor-patient interactions in which they lay out and discuss future scenarios. In all these cases, we have speakers working with global nonfictions who find it useful to turn to local instances of fictionality in order to accomplish their non-fictional purposes. Similarly, global fictions often include local instances of nonfictionality. For example, when Selzer's character narrator and Dr. Franciscus do their field trip, they travel to the nonfictional country of Honduras. In "Ten Theses about Fictionality" (see note 1), Henrik Skov Nielsen, Richard Walsh, and I contend that "Even as fictive discourse is a clear alternative to nonfictive discourse, the two are closely interrelated in continuous exchange, and so are the ways in which we engage with them" (64). My analysis of Wolff and Chast will further develop this point.

Before turning to those case studies, I want to address a couple of objections to this rhetorical conception of fictionality that some non-rhetoricians raise and another objection about distinguishing between fictionality and nonfictionality in memoirs like Wolff's and Chast's. The first comes from philosophy and particularly from epistemology. How can one draw a neat line between the actual and the invented? Given all the philosophical issues related to the question of the relation between percepts and concepts (the filters by which we interpret the world and the world itself) and all those related to the issues of what is actually "real," how can one blithely posit such a clear distinction between fictionality and nonfictionality? The objection highlights the difference between the philosophical and the rhetorical approach. For a rhetorical theorist, an interpreter's decision to take a given utterance as fictional or nonfictional is not rooted in a foundational, invariant understanding of the real and the non-real but rather in an interpretation of a speaker's intention to be using fictionality or nonfictionality. In other words, the basis for a claim that a given discourse deploys fictionality is not a bedrock belief about the clear difference between the actual and the non-actual but rather an assessment of how a given speaker views the relation between their discourse and the actual or non-actual. In this way, the decision to read an utterance as fictional is a hypothesis subject to testing and revision in the same way that other interpretations are.

The second objection comes from the domain of psychological or subjective truth. Isn't one person's fictionality another person's psychological nonfictionality? Early in her memoir, Chast draws an image of her parents as babies: they are swathed in baby bonnets and the verbal track gives their dates of birth, but she draws their adult faces, complete with their glasses. Why not say that the image conveys Chast's actual understanding of them as always already adults? From this perspective, labeling the image as an instance of "fictionality" is a misleading category error. This objection returns me to the rhetorical approach's emphasis on fictionality as an indirect means of intervening in the actual and to the import of the phrase "invents, projects, or otherwise directs [an audience] to imagine nonactual states of affairs" in the definition. If we ask where the humor of the depiction comes from, the different perspectives offer different answers. If the image is an instance of nonfictionally, a direct representation of Roz's psychological reality, then the image is not especially humorous ("this is my world"). If the image depicts an invention that indirectly gets at an actuality, then the humor comes from Chast and her audience sharing the knowledge that her parents were once actual babies and that they never simultaneously wore their adult glasses and baby bonnets. The humor, in other words, comes from the shared recognition between Chast and her audience that the visual representation is not actual but invented. At the same time, that fictionality becomes an indirect means by which Chast communicates her feeling that in some important ways her parents seem to have skipped infancy, childhood, and adolescence.

In addition, this example helps us recognize that a turn to fictionality often has its motivation in the actual rather than in the imaginative—or to put it another way, that the inventions of fictionality often depend upon an interaction of the actual and the imaginative. "Invention" is rarely, if ever, the construction of something that floats entirely free from the actual.

The third objection comes from the domain of common sense, and it applies especially to memoirs such as Wolff's and Chast's. Written years after the events—and in Wolff's case 25 years after the events—these purported nonfictional accounts must be so shot through with fictionality that the idea of distinguishing between instances of fictionality and nonfictionality should be abandoned. Memoirists take what actually happened and transform it so much that it's wiser to call their work fictions. From the perspective of rhetorical theory, this objection helps to identify the importance of considering the relation between the extratextual raw material on which memoir is based and the memoirist's shaping of that material. The rhetorical theorist acknowledges that the memoir is fully shaped—it is far from an objective recording of the raw material—but also distinguishes between shaping that claims to refer responsibly to the extratextual material and shaping that relies upon the indirections of fictionality. Furthermore, within the shaping that refers to extratextual matters, the rhetorical theorist distinguishes between accurate referentiality and lying. If someone were to show that Wolff didn't have the three close calls he tells about, or that Chast never saw her parents during their final years, then Wolff and Chast would be lying. But as long as they respect the constraints upon their shaping imposed by the extratextual raw material, the rhetorical theorist finds it both legitimate and potentially insightful to identify local instances of fictionality within their global nonfictions.

Embedded Fictionality in "Imelda"

As noted in the discussion of Imelda's progressions, Selzer uses the character narrator's imagined scenario of Franciscus going to the morgue to operate on Imelda as a crucial element of both the plot dynamics and the narratorial dynamics. The operation is the culminating event in the story of Franciscus's change, and the character narrator's imaginative reconstruction of it provides the basis for the change in his own ethical judgment of Franciscus's actions. Here I want to home in on the embedded fictionality of the scene and Selzer's specific way of handling it.

To explain why I call it embedded fictionality, I find it helpful to review rhetorical theory's proposal that the reading of fiction entails a double consciousness. Actual readers adopt two roles, that of the narrative audience who regards the characters and events as actual, and that of the authorial audience who recognizes that they are invented. Thus, in "Imelda," the authorial audience regards all the characters and events as invented, while the narrative audience regards all of them, except the character narrator's imagined scenario, as actual. Thus, the scenario is an instance of fictionality because the narrative audience recognizes it as the character narrator's invention, and it is an instance of embedded fictionality because the authorial audience recognizes it as the character narrator's invention within Selzer's invention.

I note, first, that the mimetic logic of the rest of the progression requires that the character narrator imagine the scene. Because Franciscus is stepping outside the standard boundaries of medical ethics, and because he has never treated the character narrator as a confidant, he must act alone. Selzer's challenge, then, is to make a virtue out of the necessity. He does so in two ways: (a) by having the character narrator imagine the scene through one lens rather than another; and (b) by having the character narrator be as meticulous in his imagination of the scene as Franciscus is in his surgery. Selzer could have shown the character narrator imagining the scene through the lens of his time-of-the-action judgments, a choice that would have, as I noted in Chapter 3, emphasize Franciscus's arrogance as he worked on Imelda. Instead, Selzer had the character narrator imagine the scene through the lens of his perception of Franciscus as a skilled and painstaking surgeon who has been moved in a new way by both Imelda and her mother. As I argued in Chapter 3, the character narrator's act of imagination eventually leads to the change in his ethical judgments of Franciscus, and these judgments in turn guide those of rhetorical readers.

Selzer also could have marked the character narrator's account as a fanciful flight of the character narrator's imagination, a choice that would, among other things, have shifted the focus of the scene (and perhaps the story itself) from Franciscus to the character narrator. Instead, Selzer constructs the scene to emphasize its plausibility by making the character narrator's descriptions of both the morgue and Franciscus detailed and consistent with what he knows about each. The focus then remains on Franciscus and his actions. That focus of course is appropriate for the larger progression in ways I've discussed in Chapter 3.

Fictionality in "Close Calls"

Wolff writes *In Pharaoh's Army* (note the fictionality of that title) for a general audience, 25 years after his tour of duty in the Vietnam War. He devotes his individual chapters to exploring specific episodes or general issues—chapter titles include "Thanksgiving Special," "White Man," "I Right a Wrong," and "Civilian"—even as he follows a roughly chronological order that traces his trajectory from enlisting in the Army to his experiences in Vietnam to his discharge and his start on his career as a writer. The result is a remarkable account of Wolff's struggles, his many failures, and his occasional successes in this American war effort that he now regards as at best woefully misguided and at worst an unmitigated disaster. The epigraph of the memoir, taken from Ford Madox Ford's *The Good Soldier*, gives some indication of its general purposes:

> You may well ask why I write. And yet my reasons are quite many. For it is not unusual in human beings who have witnessed the sack of a city or the falling to pieces of a people to set down what they have witnessed for the benefit of unknown heirs or of generations infinitely remote; or, if you please, just to get the sight out of their heads.

In pursuing these general purposes, Wolff strategically deploys local fictionality in various chapters in ways that significantly add to the affective and ethical dimensions of his communications. The "Close Calls" chapter is the one most relevant to Narrative Medicine because it is about mortality, and, more specifically, about experiences that lead Wolff to think about mortality—his own and that of other soldiers—in new and arresting ways.

Wolff relies on his audience's beginning their reading of the chapter with a general understanding of a close call as an experience in which what happened and what didn't happen are inextricably linked: "I could have died but I didn't." In other words, a close call is an experience in which the factuality and fictionality in the form of the counterfactual bump up against each other. By the end of the chapter, however, Wolff demonstrates that his experiences lead him to a new understanding of the phenomenon as one in which the border between the actual and the fictional is all but erased.

Wolff has his first close call after he falls asleep in his jeep in the middle of the village market only to be awakened by local citizens excitedly talking and pointing under the jeep—at a grenade with its pin pulled. Wolff gets out of the jeep but stands around gaping until his partner, Sergeant Benet, returns and takes over.

> I looked on. None of it seemed to have anything to do with me.
>
> Once the area was cleared ... we started to walk back to the battalion. Along the way I found my legs acting funny. My knees wouldn't lock; I had to lean against a wall. Sergeant Benet put his hand on my arm to steady me. Then something went slack in my belly and I felt a stream of shit pouring hotly out of me, down my legs, even into my boots. I put my head against the wall and wept for very shame.
>
> "It's all right, sir," Sergeant Benet said. "You'll be alright." ...
>
> The grenade never did go off on its own. Our ordnance disposal boys covered it with sandbags and triggered it with a dose of plastique. It was an American grenade, not some local mad bomber device. The odds of it failing like that were cruelly small—just about nonexistent, in fact.
>
> (91)

Wolff does not have the narrating-I turn toward any explicit fictionality here, but instead relies on his rhetorical readers to pick up on the implicit fictionality that is a crucial part of the event. Wolff uses the perspective of the experiencing-I who is focused on how his body reacts to the close call. That focus also prompts the question: why does he lose control of his bowels when he is out of danger? Because he is responding at some level to the counterfactual, his awareness that what is now a fictional scenario (he could have been blown up) was almost an actual one. Out of danger, yes, but almost blown to pieces. Wolff's use of the implied fictionality is more effective than a spelling out of the experiencing-I's awareness for at least two reasons. First, he can keep the issue of the degree of the experiencing-

I's conscious awareness of what almost happened open. Is Wolff's bodily response an instinctive reaction rather than the result of his consciously imagining his body spread across the town square? Rhetorical readers need not settle the question. It is far more important that Wolff registers what didn't happen at some level of consciousness. Second, Wolff's strategy of using implied fictionality guides rhetorical readers to engage more actively with the experiencing-I and to see beyond his perspective.

Wolff's account of his second close call does not use implicit or explicit fictionality but instead relies on a delayed disclosure for its effect. Consequently, I will just discuss it briefly to provide further context for Wolff's account of the third close call. Again, narrating primarily from the perspective of the experiencing-I, Wolff reports that one day, after doing the routine job of tying a big howitzer in a sling to a helicopter hovering just a few feet above him, he inexplicably watches the helicopter ascend rather than ignoring it as he usually does. As a result, he sees the howitzer fall out of the sling and hurtle to the ground, landing with such force that he "felt the shock from [his] heels to his teeth." The delayed disclosure follows: "This would not be a proper close call story if I didn't point out that the gun hit right where I'd been standing" (93). Again, Wolff guides rhetorical readers to complete the scene, and, in so doing, heightens its affective force.

Wolff's account of his third close call builds on the first two and leads to his revisionary view of the phenomenon. He relies on the exchange between fictionality and nonfictionality—and again on the inferential activity of rhetorical readers—to develop this view and make it persuasive.

In this experience, Wolff and another soldier, Keith Young, are standing next to each other among a group at headquarters listening to situation reports on the radio. As they listen, the ranking officer, General Lance, places his hand on Keith's shoulder. Thus, when a sudden call for help comes in over the radio, General Lance turns to him and says, "Well, Keith, what do you think?" (94). Wolff narrates the consequences:

> Keith got killed later that afternoon. I never heard what the circum-
> stances were, only that he got shot in the stomach … .
> Everything marched in lockstep from [General Lance's arbitrary deci-
> sion to stand to Keith's right]. If he had stood between us, it would have
> been my shoulder the hand fell on, the other hand being occupied with
> his curved, fragrant, fatherly pipe. It would have been me receiving the
> father's thoughtless blessing touch, me to whom he turned, me to whom
> he put the kindly question that had only one answer.
>
> (95)

In this passage, Wolff offers another variation on the exchange between nonfictionality and fictionality. Wolff goes beyond the implicit fictionality of the first close call to this projection of what could so easily have happened if General Lance had stood between Keith and himself. Although this close call does not involve the immediate threat to Wolff's life that the first and second ones did, it does involve his and his audience's imagining what didn't happen. Wolff's reflection on the thin line between what did and didn't happen leads him to thematize all three experiences:

> In a world where the most consequential things happen by chance, or from unfathomable causes, you don't look to reason for help. You consort with mysteries. You encourage yourself with charms, omens, rites of propriation. Without your knowledge, the bottom-line cave-man belief in blood sacrifice, one life buying another, begins to steal into your bones. How could it not? All around you people are killed: soldiers on both sides, farmers, teachers, mothers, fathers, schoolgirls, nurses, your friends—but not you. They have been killed instead of you. This observation is unavoidable. So, in time, is the corollary, implicit in the word *instead:* in place of. They have been killed in place of you—in your place … . It's the close call you have to keep escaping from, the unending doubt that you have the right to your own life. It's the corruption suffered by everyone who lives on, that henceforth they must wonder at the reason and probe its justice.
>
> (96–97)

The experience of close calls, in other words, leads to the breakdown of the normal relation between the actual and the non-actual. In actuality, all these others (farmers, teachers, etc.) have been killed by the circumstances that led to their deaths, most of which have nothing to do with Wolff. But Wolff's experience of close calls makes it impossible to hold on to that actuality, to keep the fictionality that they have been killed "instead of" him in the realm of the non-actual. That impossibility in turn means that the close call is not a single, bounded event but an ongoing incessant narrative: "It's the close call you have to keep escaping from." Wolff's experiences of close calls lead to his almost erasing the distinction between the actual and the fictional.

Wolff closes out the chapter with a turn to explicit fictionality that exemplifies his thematizing of the close call. Wolff's first move is to recall the one extended encounter he had with Keith Young. Both men were going to Hong Kong for R&R, and Keith was excited about a great deal on allegedly high-quality suits he could get from a tailor there. Wolff went along and watched Keith getting fit for an extensive wardrobe. Wolff got caught up in the excitement and ordered some suits of his own. Wolff rounds out the account as follows:

> We hit a few clubs that night and he couldn't stop talking about what a great deal he'd gotten. And that was the first thought I had when I heard that he'd been killed. What about all those clothes? It was a gasp

of a thought, completely instinctual, without malice or irony. All those clothes waiting for him—they seemed somehow an irrefutable argument for his survival … .

Wolff then ends with the explicit fictionality:

> I sometimes tried to imagine other men wearing Keith's suits, but I couldn't bring the images to life. What I see instead is a dark closet with all his clothes hanging in a row. Someone opens the closet door, looks at them for a time, and closes the door again.
>
> (98)

This last sentence invites the question, "who is the someone who opens the door?" One plausible answer is "a member of Keith's family," and that answer points to Wolff's inability to imagine the suits on someone else and to his effort to communicate something of the effect of Keith's death on those close to him. But the previous two sentences make "Tobias Wolff" another plausible answer. Since Wolff imagines the whole scenario, he inevitably imagines himself opening the door, staring at the suits, and then closing it, a sequence that reminds him yet again of how close he came to losing his life. Both answers, in combination with the shift to the present tense and thus the occasion of the telling 25 years after the events, indicate that Wolff remains haunted by Keith's death. In this way, this final turn to explicit fictionality clinches Wolff's defamiliarization of the close call, the way it practically erases the border between the actual and the non-actual and the way its effects continue beyond the moment of its occurrence. These effects deepen the ethical and affective dimensions of his defamiliarization.

Fictionality and Nonfictionality in Chast's *Can't We Talk?*

In keeping with the discussion in the last chapter, I will focus my analysis of Chast's *Can't We Talk?* on the relation between fictionality and nonfictionality as it gets mapped on to the relation between the verbal and the visual. Several kinds of mapping are possible. Both the verbal and the visual can be nonfictional or fictional; the verbal can be fictional and the visual nonfictional, and vice versa. Furthermore, within a visual use of fictionality, dialogue/thought can be nonfictional. Similarly, within a visual use of nonfictionality, dialogue/thought can be fictional. In addition, within a visual use of fictionality, dialogue/thought can also be fictional. These relationships should become clearer as we look at specific excerpts. In addition to looking at the various uses of (non)fictionality within the verbal and visual tracks, I shall also pay attention to how they function in relation to Chast's overall purposes.

At this point, we can supplement Chapter 9's commentary on Chast's depiction of the relation between clock time and subjective time (see Figure 9.10) by noting that the sequence of images of the clock progresses from nonfictionality to increasing fictionality along both the verbal and visual tracks. This thicker description also points to the ease with which rhetorical readers often negotiate the exchange between fictionality and nonfictionality.

Figure 10.1 shows Chast using fictionality within both the verbal and the visual tracks of communication as she advances a thematic point. There are some important nuances to the interactions here. First, the verbal track deploys embedded fictionality: Chast makes a serious proposal about changing the actualities of end-of-life care, even as that proposal depends on her invention of the alternative. (In this way, Chast's use of embedded fictionality has one less layer than Selzer's use of it in "Imelda": he embeds the character narrator's imagined scene of Franciscus in the morgue within a fictional short story, while Chast embeds her projection within her nonfictional memoir.) Within Chast's verbal track, the link between the actual and the invented is tighter than, say, the one operating in the visual image, since that one skips over any embedding and places Elizabeth in a fictional temporal and spatial realm. That use of fictionality adds humor to the interaction, but together the verbal and the visual powerfully communicate Chast's thematic point about changing the norms for end-of-life care.

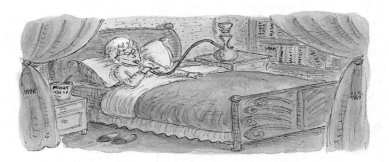

Figure 10.1 Extreme palliative care

Second, the fictionality of the visual track, by putting Elizabeth in a non-actual spatial and temporal frame, foregrounds the thematic component of her character: she represents the larger class of people who are "done." Chast uses Elizabeth's mimetic character both to add humor to the page—the Elizabeth depicted in the rest of the memoir is not one to be taking drugs—and to highlight the distance from current practices to her proposed ones. But the image adds to Chast's case because this Elizabeth is far more serene than the one she depicts in the rest of the memoir.

Figures 10.2 and 10.3 are examples of verbal nonfictionality interacting with visual fictionality. In the visual images, Chast draws on well-known fictional figures, the Grim Reaper, and the screamer in Edvard Munch's *The Scream*, to create some remarkable effects that contribute to her larger purposes.

In Figure 10.2 Chast overlays Munch's figure on her own portrait as a way to capture her distress at the news that her mother had fallen and been taken to the hospital in the middle of the night. Chast's overlay demonstrates the way in which fictionality can offer a "double exposure" (see Nielsen, Phelan, and Walsh) of the fictional and nonfictional: the image is a version of Chast, but it is also a version of the screamer. In such double exposures the link between the actual and invented is very tight. With this image, Chast both captures Roz's deep distress at the news and, much like Engelberg in her "Everything Is My Enemy" splash page (discussed in Chapter 9), indicates that the artist has a perspective on what's happening that the experiencing-I does not.

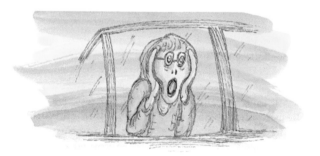

It was a Life Alert sort of person. Duh. My mother and father were at the emergency room at Maimonides Hospital in Brooklyn. An ambulance had brought them both. My father couldn't be left alone, and he didn't know how to drive.

Figure 10.2 Double exposure: The Scream

In Figure 10.3 The Grim Reaper sits on the couch in Elizabeth and George's living room, not only comically signaling his comfort in their place but also adding another dimension to Roz's affective response. Not only is she stuck with the tedious task of dealing with what her parents have left behind, but she will have to do it in the presence of this unpleasant companion.

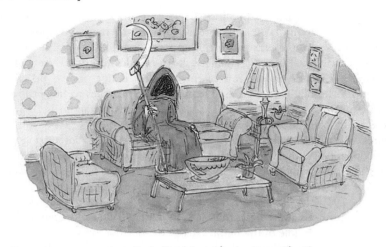

I was aggravated that they hadn't dealt with their accumulations, back when they had the ability to do so. That instead, when they decided to leave, they simply packed a couple of little bags and walked out, leaving me the task of cleaning out their apartment.

Figure 10.3 A visit from the Grim Reaper

Figures 10.1, 10.2, and 10.3 as well as some reflection on Wolff's "Close Calls" provide the basis for a clearer understanding of the activity of rhetorical readers in responding to local fictionality in global nonfiction. These uses of local fictionality do not generate a narrative audience. In other words, in constructing the exchanges between fictionality and nonfictionality in their memoirs, neither Wolff nor Chast generates the double consciousness in their readers that Selzer and other writers of global fictions do (characters are real and autonomous actors; characters are invented constructs). Instead, they ask rhetorical readers to recognize the move to fictionality and seek the point of the indirect communication. In Figure 10.1, for example, Chast does not ask her rhetorical readers to buy into the illusion that Elizabeth with her hookah pipe is real in the way Selzer asks his narrative audience to regard Imelda as real. Instead, Chast flaunts the fictionality of her image for her rhetorical readers, inviting them to see how her invention supports her nonfictional recommendations about handling pain at the end-of-life. With this understanding in mind, let's look at a few more striking examples of Chast's use of fictionality. The ones I choose are connected to the resources of plot, character, and temporality.

In Figure 10.4, we can see Chast embedding fictionality within non-fictionality as she introduces the larger issue of a plot for her parents' last years.

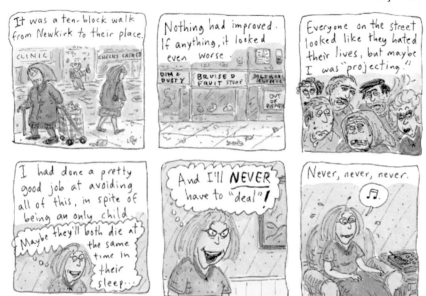

Figure 10.4 Wishful thinking

Chast projects a wish-fulfillment plot, but she has already given her audience enough information to indicate that her wish will not be fulfilled. In this way, the embedded fictionality gives a poignant quality to the situation of the experiencing-Roz, because rhetorical readers recognize the gap between the plot Roz desires and the unfolding plot of Chast's memoir.

In Figure 10.5, we see Chast using the interaction between verbal non-fictionality and visual fictionality to highlight Roz's realizations about the actual plot she is living through. The visual fictionality depicts one master plot for the end-of-life. The fictional Old Mrs. McGillicuddy (and note how "old" moves from an adjective to her first name across the panels, part of Chast's equating her identity with her age and marital status) dies relatively painlessly within three or four weeks of becoming ill. The verbal nonfictionality provides the sharp contrast: "the middle panel was a lot more painful, humiliating, long-lasting, complicated, and hideously expensive." Among other things, the interaction works in the service of Chast's thematizing of her experience: the new under-standing of the middle panel applies not just to her but to so many like her.

In Figures 10.6, 10.7, and 10.8, we see how Chast uses the exchange between fictionality and nonfictionality to depict the characters of Elizabeth and George. Figure 10.6 visually literalizes Elizabeth's metaphor of George "walking around with his feelers out" even as the verbal track conveys his typical thoughts and reactions ("was that an insult?"). In this way, Chast sets up a close exchange between fictionality and nonfictionality that humorously, sympathetically, and efficiently depicts a key component of George's character.

Here's what I used to think happened at "the end":

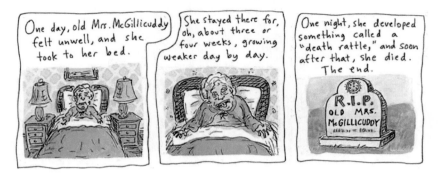

What I was starting to understand was that the middle panel was a lot more painful, humiliating, long-lasting, complicated, and hideously expensive. My parents had been in pretty good health for

Figure 10.5 The last days of Mrs. McGillicuddy

And, more important, he was kind and sensitive. He knew that my mother had a terrible temper, and that she could be overpowering. She had a thick skin. He, like me, did not. She often accused my father of "walking around with his feelers out."

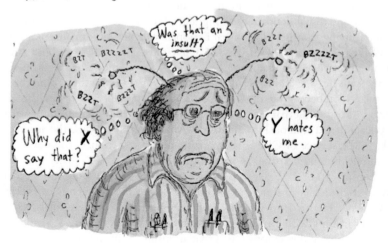

Figure 10.6 George with his "feelers out"

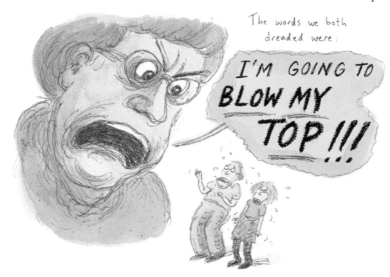

Figure 10.7 A Blast from Chast

She was sleeping a lot. She wasn't eating much. She'd wake up and Goodie would give her an Ensure, and she'd go back to sleep. However, even at this point, she looked disconcertingly sturdy. When my father was "at the end," he looked frail-almost skeletal. My mother looked... robust.

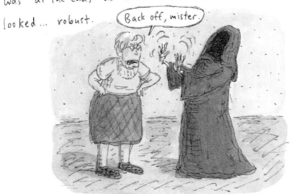

Figure 10.8 Resisting the Grim Reaper

Figure 10.7 uses the visual image to construct the metaphor of Elizabeth as a large, looming figure—a human storm. Along with depictions of her mother's own announcements that she would give someone a "Blast from Chast," the page effectively captures Elizabeth's dominance over Roz and her father. Figure 10.8 shows Chast building on these depictions of her parents' characters as she uses the visual fictionality to show Elizabeth making the Grim Reaper back off and the verbal nonfictionality to draw the contrast with her father's condition and behavior at the end-of-life.

Figures 10.9, 10.10, and 10.11 show how Chast uses fictionality in the representation of her own character as experiencing-I. In Figure 10.9,

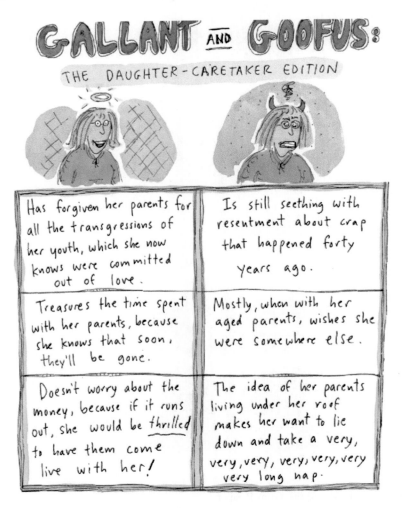

Figure 10.9 Roz as Gallant and Goofus

hospital every few months for x-rays. I didn't walk until I was
18 months old - about half a year later than average.

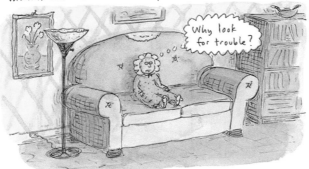

It was determined that there was nothing wrong with me. Nevertheless,
I was probably not a fun baby. I had one cold after another,
and from the time I could speak, one anxiety after another. I
was my father's daughter, not my mother's.

Figure 10.10 Not a fun baby

another good example of the double exposure that the turn to fictionality
sometimes provides, Chast adapts the fictional trope of Goofus and Gallant
from *Highlights for Children* magazine and sets up a remarkable relation
between fictionality and nonfictionality: in each column, Chast highlights
extremes, a move that indicates that she is combining fictionality and nonfictionality. In other words, she is neither wholly Gallant nor wholly
Goofus—even if she does not try to specify the exact nature of the blend.
Chast's openness about being at least partially "Goofus" and admitting her
flaws—ones that her rhetorical readers will find understandable—adds to her
admirable overall ethos.

In Figures 10.10 and 10.11, Chast uses the exchange between fictionality
and nonfictionality to convey her sense of Roz's position within her family.
Reflecting on her childhood struggles in the nonfictional verbal narration in
Figure 10.10, she links her character with her father's, but the fictional
temporality of the thought bubble gives her a kind of self-insight and wit
that rhetorical readers never see George possess.

Figure 10.11 is part of the sequence of family photographs that I discussed
in Chapter 9. Chast adds two twists to this one: the image of Roz clearly
marks her as the unhappy one; and the fictionality of the humorous
thought bubble, an addition by the artist at the time of the telling, further
highlights the distance between Roz and her parents and points toward
her pre-teen restlessness.

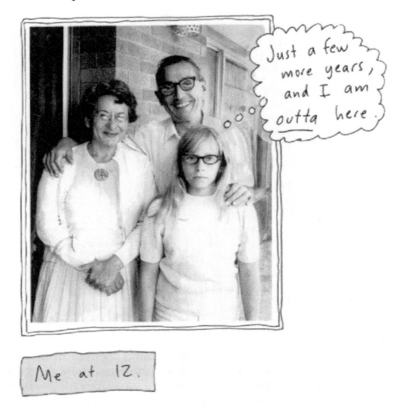

Figure 10.11 Elizabeth, George, and a restless Roz

Stepping back from this commentary on particular images, I note that Chast's practice provides the basis for an initial—and partial—taxonomy of kinds of fictionality within a graphic memoir. This taxonomy focuses on the visual side but it's relevant to the verbal side as well.

- Straight invention (sometimes of the counterfactual): Elizabeth with the hookah pipe.
- Use of an established fictional trope: The Grim Reaper.
- Adaptation of a trope (with double exposure): The Scream, Goofus and Gallant.
- Literalizing a metaphor: "Feelers out."
- Embedded imaginings.
- Temporal play between fictionality and thought/speech.

As I hope the analysis shows, there is no one-to-one correspondence between any kind of fictionality and its effects. Instead, the effects depend on the specific deployment of the kind in its particular context. In addition, Chast demonstrates the power of overt fictionality in nonfiction: rather than constructing a narrative audience and asking it to buy into the illusion of fiction, she asks rhetorical readers to share both the invention and the knowledge that it's invented. This strategy constructs a more direct relation between author and audience than we find in fiction and contributes a great deal to Chast's construction of her own ethos. Without her uses of fictionality, Chast's memoir would be far different—and, I would suggest, a far less powerful narrative.

Finally, Chast's memoir provides a telling example of how fictionality can be a powerful resource to come to terms with the often-difficult experiences associated with caring for others at the end of their lives. Chast demonstrates that fictionality can provide perspective, salutary humor, and compelling ways of dealing with the realities of such situations. In capturing her own experiences in such a distinctive and engaging manner, Chast provides a model that others can adapt to the specific exigencies of their own experiences.

Opening Out

Fictionality is a valuable resource for caregivers and patients, precisely because it is an indirect rather than direct means of engaging with the actual. They can take advantage of its indirection to conduct conversations that would be much more difficult if they were restricted to nonfictionality. To a patient with a scary diagnosis, a caregiver can say, "I can't make firm predictions, but we can together consider some hypothetical scenarios." Because the caregiver explicitly marks the scenarios as instances of fictionality, the patient is more likely to engage with them. After that engagement, the caregiver and patient can then shift back to the actual and agree upon a treatment plan.[2]

Caregivers and patients can also use the indirectness of fictionality to make their storytelling more vivid and effective. To engage in a little fictionality myself, imagine Wolff telling the story of his third close call to a therapist. If the therapist were any good, they would neither object to Wolff's departures from the actual nor seek to correct his conflation of fictionality and nonfictionality. Instead, the therapist would recognize that Wolff's fictionality already demonstrates remarkable self-insight, and they could go from there. Few caregivers or patients, of course, are as accomplished at storytelling as Wolff, but his performance can give each group the confidence that the turn to fictionality can enhance rather than impede their communications.

Overstanding Prompt

Respond to this claim: Wolff's "Close Calls," despite its effectiveness on its own terms, suffers from its failure to go beyond those terms and critique the problems that stem from the masculinity underlying norms about how soldiers should behave during times of war. These norms operate in Wolff's consternation at his body's reaction to the first close call, in his implicit pride in escaping the howitzer in the second close call, and in his response to Keith Young's death. Make the case for this position and then respond to it, agreeing or disagreeing, in whole or in part, and giving warrants for your response.

Springboarding Prompts

Rewrite the story of Wolff's third close call from Keith Young's perspective (up to the point of his responding to Colonel Lance's suggestion/order) and include at least one instance of local fictionality.

Convert the story of one of Wolff's close calls into a graphic narrative.

If you've had a close call, tell the story about it—in comics or prose—and include at least one instance of local fictionality.

Tell the story—in comics or prose—of a challenging experience you had when you were far from home and include at least one example of local fictionality.

Tell your version of Chast's story—in comics or prose—about "Old Mrs. McGillicuddy" and include at least one instance of local fictionality.

Tell a short fictional illness narrative—in comics or prose—and then identify any instances of nonfictionality within it.

Notes

1 The foundational text for this line of thinking is Richard Walsh's *A Rhetoric of Fictionality* (2007). In "Ten Theses about Fictionality" (2015), Walsh collaborated with Henrik Skov Nielsen and me to elaborate on the approach. The collection, *Fictionality in Literature: Core Concepts Revisited*, co-edited by the three of us and Lasse Gammelgaard, Stefan Iversen, Louise Brix Jakobsen, and Simona Zetterberg Nielsen (2022) offers further expansion of the approach.
2 I owe this point to a conversation with Dr. Kathy Kirkland, a specialist in palliative care,

Works Cited

Chast, Roz. *Can't We Talk About Something More Pleasant?* London: Bloomsbury, 2014.
Coetzee, J.M. *Scenes from Provincial Life: Boyhood, Youth, Summertime.* New York: Penguin, 2012.
Cohn, Dorrit. *The Distinction of Fiction.* Baltimore, MD: Johns Hopkins Press, 1999.
Nielsen, Henrik Skov, James Phelan, and Richard Walsh. "Ten Theses About Fictionality." *Narrative* 23, 1 (2015): 61–73.
Phelan, James. *Narrative as Rhetoric.* Columbus, OH: Ohio State University Press, 1996.

Phelan, James. *Somebody Telling Somebody Else: Toward a Rhetorical Poetics of Narrative.* Columbus, OH: Ohio State University Press, 2017.

Selzer, Richard. "Imelda." In *The Doctor Stories*, 83–97. New York: Picador, 1998.

Walsh, Richard. *A Rhetoric of Fictionality*. Columbus, OH: The Ohio State University Press, 2007.

Wolff, Tobias. *In Pharoah's Army*. New York: Knopf, 1994.

Zetterberg-Nielsen, Henrik , Richard Walsh, Stefan Iversen, Simona Zetterberg-Nielsen, Louise Brix Jacobsen, Lasse Raaby Gammelgaard, and James Phelan. *Fictionality in Literature: Core Concepts Revisited*. Columbus, OH: The Ohio State University Press, 2022.

11 Rhetorical Narrative Medicine Workshops
Understanding, Overstanding, and Springboarding

Now that we have worked through a rhetorical approach to the major resources of narrative, a task that has emphasized the challenges and rewards of close reading/careful listening with glances toward the steps of overstanding and springboarding, I close this book by sketching a template for conducting and participating in Rhetorical Narrative Medicine workshops. These workshops can be stand-alone sessions or they can be integrated into term-length courses. They can be productive for those new to Narrative Medicine and for those who want to refresh their knowledge of it.

This template describes a process with the three steps of understanding (based on close reading), overstanding (assessing the results of understanding), and springboarding (seeking connections between the understanding or overstanding and other matters of readerly interest). This commitment to process also involves putting a premium on the learning that arises from the exchange of ideas among workshop participants and from individual participants having the opportunity to write out their own thoughts. Consequently, in this chapter, I will shift from my previous practice of carrying out my own rhetorical readings to one of posing questions and offering prompts for discussion or writing across its three segments. Within the springboarding segment, I will propose some prompts specifically for written responses. I describe a workshop focused on Jesmyn Ward's remarkable nonfiction narrative, "On Witness and Respair: A Personal Tragedy Followed by Pandemic," published in *Vanity Fair* in September of 2020.

As noted in Chapter 2, rhetorical readers engaging in understanding seek consensus about an author's narrative purposes and their ways of achieving them, but rhetorical readers engaging in overstanding and springboarding do not. As a result, the progression of a narrative workshop will initially seek consensus and then encourage participants to express and explore their differences. Overstanding and springboarding are concerned with what individual readers—or different groups of readers—do AFTER the work of understanding, and rhetorical theory expects and encourages readers, because of their different identities, experiences, and interests, to

DOI: 10.4324/9781003018865-11

at least sometimes do different things. To put this point another way, both overstanding and springboarding are more free-form activities than understanding, and they welcome the different responses of different readers—and the dialogues that can follow from the articulation of those differences. Furthermore, the goal of such dialogues is not primarily to reduce such differences (though if participants move toward consensus, that's typically a good thing). Instead, the goal is to increase the participants' understanding (!) of each other's positions—what their sources and consequences are likely to be. To achieve that goal, participants need to be open to where the discussions of initial differences may lead. For these reasons, I will not specify or predict any outcomes of overstanding Ward's narrative or springboarding from it. Narrative workshops are better when their outcomes are not scripted in advance.

Stage One: Toward an Understanding of "On Witness and Respair"

As I hope the previous chapters demonstrate, a rhetorical analyst can move toward understanding by proposing a hypothesis about an author's purposes, identifying the especially salient resources used to achieve those purposes, and then doing close readings of the authorial deployments of those resources. A Narrative Medicine workshop can productively follow this sequence, though, for the sake of efficiency, the workshop leader might want to begin by proposing a hypothesis about the author's purposes. For the sake of efficiency here, I will take that route.

Purposes: Ward's purposes are both general and specific. She tells the nonfictional story of her husband's death from COVID-19 in January 2020 at the age of 33 and then traces her responses to his death through her responses to the pandemic and to the Black Lives Matter (BLM) protests that followed the killing of George Floyd in May 2020. Ward's general purpose is to explore the connections between individual experience and social and political history. Her specific purposes involve connecting her personal tragedy to the experiences of others who are responding to grief and suffering brought on by the pandemic and by systemic racism so that she can find for herself, and offer to others, reasons for realistic hope. She encapsulates this idea in her portmanteau "respair," which blends "despair" with "repair" and "respire" (more on this portmanteau below).

Resources: Since Ward draws on all the resources we have discussed in significant ways, workshop participants face a happy problem: there won't be time to discuss all of the resources, but there are no bad choices. After raising some questions about the occasion of Ward's telling, I'll organize my observations and questions around the progression but bring in other resources when they become especially relevant. Again, I'm offering an illustration of one way to proceed. Singling out other passages or putting the main focus on other resources would generate other observations and questions.

Observations and Questions about the Occasion

In September 2020, the United States was still struggling to respond to the COVID-19 pandemic that had caused the illness and death of so many people since the beginning of the year. On May 25, 2020, Minneapolis police officer Derek Chauvin murdered George Floyd, sparking international demonstrations in support of the BLM movement. In addition, businesses, hospitals, educational institutions and many other entities had pledged that they would give new attention to issues of social justice. How does this context influence your understanding of what it means for Ward to publish this piece when she did? What does the context suggest about how it might be received? How does its publication in *Vanity Fair* rather than, say, *The New Yorker*, or *The New York Times Magazine* influence your understanding of it? If Ward were to publish it now—that is, at the time you're reading this book—how would that affect your understanding of it? What differences do you see between the occasion of its telling and the occasion of your reading it?

Observations and Questions about the Progression

Ward's first sentence is "My beloved died in January" and her last is "*We here.*" The first sentence clearly introduces an instability (in the narrative and in her life), but does the last achieve a resolution, and, if so, how?

What are the main segments of the plot dynamics? Are there markers of stages in the plot? One hypothesis worth discussing and perhaps refining: there are three main movements, which also correspond to ways in which Ward organizes the temporality of her experiences.

1   January 2020, the month in which her husband dies, and her grief begins. That grief functions as the major instability in the first two segments of her piece.
2   March to June, the months in which the significant complications of the experiencing-I's grieving include her newfound awareness of the cause of her husband's death: COVID-19.
3   June to August, the months during which her grief intersects with her responses to the BLM protests. During this segment Ward shifts toward a more essayistic mode as she introduces a second major instability, the condition of being Black in America.

If that's a working hypothesis of the plot dynamics, what are the key features of the narratorial dynamics? How does Ward handle the shifts from the narrating-I's perspective at the time of the telling to the experiencing-I's perspective at the time of the action?

Ward's narratee is someone who does not have prior knowledge of Ward's family but does know about the pandemic, the murder of George

Floyd, and the BLM protests. Do you feel addressed by Ward, or do you feel that you are observing her address some other narratee? If the latter, then who?

Looking more closely at the first stage of the progression, we see that, after that arresting first sentence, Ward does not immediately tell about how her husband died but instead sketches the mimetic component of his character: he was a devoted, self-sacrificing, and loving husband and father ("One of my favorite places in the world was beside him, under his warm arm, the color of deep, dark river water"). Returning then to the how, Ward reports that she, he, and their two children became ill with what they thought was the flu and that everyone got better except her husband. After he "panted: *Can't. Breathe*," she took him to the hospital, where he was put on a ventilator. But his organs failed, and he died within 15 hours of being admitted. At that point, the experiencing-I sinks into "hot, wordless grief."

What are the readerly dynamics in this stretch of the narrative? What are your ethical judgments and affective responses to the mimetic portrait of Ward's husband? To his death? Do you feel the emotions associated with the word Ward uses in her title, tragedy? Do those emotions—or whichever ones you feel—apply both to the experiencing-I and her husband or to just one? At this stage, is there anything that might be called catharsis, or any movement toward a resolution of the experiencing-I's grief? Does Ward's act of telling itself appear to be therapeutic in any way?

In the second movement of the progression, Ward greatly complicates the global instability, as she indicates that the experiencing-I's feelings of loss continue unabated: "The absence of my Beloved echoed in every room" of their house, and "My grief bloomed into depression," even as she struggled to write her novel about "the hell of chattel slavery in the mid-1800s." At the same time, learning about the pandemic revises the experiencing-I's understanding of the cause of her husband's death, and that revision in turn evokes new fears about the pandemic's ongoing effects. Ward expresses those fears in one long, extraordinary sentence:

> During the pandemic, I couldn't bring myself to leave the house, terrified I would find myself standing in the doorway of an ICU room, watching the doctors press their whole weight on the chest of my mother, my sisters, my children, terrified of the lurch of their feet, the lurch that accompanies each press that restarts the heart, the jerk of their pale, tender soles, terrified of the frantic prayer without intention that keens through the mind, the prayer for life that one says in the doorway, the prayer I never want to say again, the prayer that dissolves midair when the hush-click-hush-click of the ventilator drowns it, terrified of the terrible commitment at the heart of me that reasons that if the person I love has to endure this, then the least I can do is stand there, the least I can do is witness, the least I can do is tell them over and over again, aloud, *I love you. We love you. We ain't going nowhere.*

So many resources to contemplate here. What is Ward doing with time? How does she blend singulative and iterative narration? How about order, or more specifically, what is the relation she sets up among past, present, and future? How does that temporality affect what she is doing with perspective? What of the opposition between the spatial frames of house and hospital? How many voices are here, and how do they relate to each other? Who is the "we" in the last lines?

The passage also includes an instance of local fictionality in the form of a double exposure of the experiencing-I's memory of her husband and her projection of that scene onto possible others. Does that local fictionality enhance or detract from the scene? Why?

This passage is the first time that Ward uses the title word "witness" in the body of the essay. What weight does she give it here? What do you make of its connection with "I love you"?

As for readerly dynamics, how does Ward orchestrate the interaction of affect and ethics? Are rhetorical readers feeling the tragic emotions of pity and fear more deeply, or does the way Ward's vision extends beyond her husband and her immediate family blunt those responses?

Ward begins the third segment with the experiencing-I's responses to her cousin's telling her about George Floyd's killing:

> *Cuz*, I said, *I think you told me this story before.*
> *I think I wrote it.*
> I swallowed sour.

Here Ward suggests that her cousin's news will just add to the experiencing-I's depression. But then the news of the protests brings in the new instability and Ward's reflections on it: the condition of being Black in America. The experiencing-I's first response to the news is to weep, as "The revelation that Black Americans were not alone in this, that others around the world believed that Black Lives Matter broke something in me, some immutable belief I'd carried with me my whole life." This belief is that "Black lives have the same value as a plow horse or a grizzled donkey." Ward testifies that the belief "beat like another heart" throughout her life, and she relates harrowing incidents in her life or in the lives of family members that reinforced the belief.

Ward then moves into this broader reflection:

> My people knew [that Black lives were devalued], and we fought it, but we were convinced we would fight this reality alone, fight until we could no more, until we were in the ground, bones moldering, headstones overgrown above in the world where our children and children's children still fought, still yanked against the noose, the forearm, the starvation and redlining and rape and enslavement and murder and choked out: *I can't breathe.* They would say: *I can't breathe.* *I can't breathe.*

How does the new instability relate to the one about her grief? How is Ward handling time here? Why would she, after signaling a turning point with her declaration that the protests broke her "immutable belief," not immediately follow through by addressing the significance of that change? Why return to the past instead? Does it make sense to think of this passage as a pause in the forward movement of the plot? Do you think it helps to suggest that Ward begins to blend essay-like exposition and reflection here?

Again, voice becomes salient. How does Ward handle the relation between first-person singular and first-person plural? How does the repetition of "I can't breathe" link with her husband's voicing of "*Can't breathe*" just before he goes to the hospital? Does that link suggest anything about the relation between the instability about grief and the one about the protests?

What of readerly dynamics? What are the layers of affective response generated by the textual dynamics, especially the movement between the present change (the breaking of the immutable belief) and the references to the past? What is the relation among such responses as hope, sorrow, and empathy?

In the penultimate step of the progression, Ward offers an explicit discussion of witnessing:

> I cried in wonder each time I saw protest around the world because I recognized the people ... I recognized their action for what it was: witness. Even now, each day, they witness.
>
> They witness injustice.
>
> They witness this America, this country that gaslit us for 400 fucking years.
>
> Witness that my state, Mississippi, waited until 2013 to ratify the 13th Amendment ... .
>
> Witness Black people, Indigenous people, so many poor brown people, lying on beds in frigid hospitals, gasping our last breaths with COVID-riddled lungs, rendered flat by undiagnosed underlying conditions, triggered by years of food deserts, stress, and poverty ... .
>
> They witness our fight too, the quick jerk of our feet, see our hearts lurch to beat again in our art and music and work and joy. How revelatory that others witness our battles and stand up. They go out in the middle of a pandemic, and they march.
>
> I sob, and the rivers of people run in the streets.

How does Ward connect her previous account of the experiencing-I's witnessing in the ICU with the witnessing of those "who witness our battles ... and march"? Does the experiencing-I join in their witnessing, or does she remain an observer of it? What is the connection between the experiencing-I's sobbing and the "rivers of people" running in the streets? More generally, how do these complications of the second instability of the BLM protests relate to the initial instability of grief about her husband's death? How do the new emotions of the experiencing-I—anger and disgust and release—relate to her grief?

How do all these things, plus Ward's handling of time (past and present) and space (the expansion of the frame to include the world and then the contraction of it to "frigid hospitals"), shed light on the second key word of her title, "respair"? The portmanteau draws on "despair," "repair," and, given the references to COVID-19, ventilators, and gasping, "respire." Does Ward seem to give more weight to any one of these source words than the others?

The final move of the progression refers back to the scene of the experiencing-I's witnessing in the ICU.

> When my beloved died, a doctor told me: *The last sense to go is hearing.*
> *When someone is dying, they lose sight and smell and taste and touch. They*
> *even forget who they are. But in the end, they hear you.*
>   I hear you.
>   I hear you.
>   You say:
>   *I love you.*
>   *We love you.*
>   *We ain't going nowhere.*
>   I hear you say:
>   *We here.*

What happens to perspective at this point? Is it fair to say that Ward merges the perspectives of the experiencing-I and the narrating-I? What happens to the referents of I, you, and we as the passage progresses? Is it plausible to read the "I" as both Ward and her husband, and "you" as both her husband and the BLM protesters? And "we" as all three? How do those answers affect an understanding of voice? And of the force of the repetition of lines from the earlier scene? Is Ward creating another double exposure of fictionality (her husband expressing his love to her on his deathbed—or perhaps on hers) and nonfictionality (her expressing her love to him in those moments)? How does this ending relate to the thematics of witnessing and respair that the previous movements of the progression have been developing? What is the effect of concluding with a phrase, "*We here,*" that was not in the earlier scene? How does the pun on "here/hear" connect with the concept of witnessing as involving seeing and testifying?

As for readerly dynamics, Ward certainly guides her rhetorical readers to affirm the extraordinary witnessing she represents, but how does that ethical affirmation connect with the layering of affective responses? Is Ward inviting her audience to experience their own sense of respair? Again, is Ward giving more weight to "repair" than "despair"?

Stage Two: Overstanding

A few reminders from the discussion in Chapter 2: overstanding is about stepping back from understanding and assessing it. Overstanding can be positive, negative, and mixed. It often leads back into understanding, as one seeks to ground the assessment in details of the rhetorical communication.

Here are some prompts for overstanding Ward's narrative, the first several of which can be easily adapted for other narratives. These prompts can be used to generate group discussion or short writing responses by each participant:

What do you find most impressive about "On Witness and Respair"?

What do you find most challenging to your ideas, beliefs, assumptions, attitudes, and behavior?

If Ward came to you with the narrative before publication and asked you to edit it, what advice would you give her?

Does Ward successfully capture a distinct emotion with her concept of "respair"? If so, how significant do you find it? If not, then how does your answer affect your overall response to her narrative?

How is respair related to resilience? Would resilience work as well as respair as a key term/concept in Ward's narrative?

Circling back to the issue of occasion: how do you think reading Ward's narrative when it came out in September 2020 was different from reading it today? Has it gained power over time, or has it become dated? Be open to saying that some parts have gained power and others have faded.

Stage Three: Springboarding

Writing or discussion prompts:

Compare and contrast Ward's narrative with Oates's "Widow's First Year" and "Hospice/Honeymoon."

How would you extend Ward's testimony about the power of witnessing to other contexts?

How can Ward's narrative be helpful to those dealing with their own personal tragedies?

Writing prompts:

Write a short narrative about Ward's husband's end-of-life experiences from his perspective. Start with his diagnosis and end shortly before his death.

Write your own pandemic-related narrative (fictional, nonfictional, or auto-fictional).

Write about a time when you were in a situation that made you especially conscious of your racial identity.

Write about events in your family's history whose effects you and/or others in your family still feel to this day.

Write about a time when you were fearful.

Write about a time when you were inspired by the actions of others.

Write about a time when you felt a strong sense of being part of a group that was more than the sum of its individual members.

Again, this template should be adjusted to meet the possibilities and constraints of particular workshops. What's most important for the success of any workshop is the investment of the participants in engaging with the selected narrative and with each other. Such engagements, when they include attention to understanding, overstanding, and springboarding, can contribute substantially to the participants' knowing-that and knowing-how.

Works Cited

Ward, Jesmyn. "On Witness and Respair: A Personal Tragedy Followed by Pandemic." *Vanity Fair*, 1 September 2020. www.vanityfair.com/culture/2020/08/jesmyn-ward-on-husbands-death-and-grief-during-covid (Accessed 11 February 2022.)

Epilog
Resolution, Reconfiguration, Farewell

Just as the Preface turned a rhetorical lens on the project of this book, this epilog will look at the previous 11 chapters through the lens of progression, and more specifically through the constructs of resolution, reconfiguration, and farewell. On the one hand, I am acutely aware that I cannot claim that the book has achieved a resolution in which all possible questions about a rhetorical prescription for Narrative Medicine have been asked and answered. I acknowledge that (a) the theoretical treatments of the resources could be (even) more detailed; (b) the analyses of their uses in each chapter could be (even) more extensive; (c) even more resources could be analyzed, as a review of the list in Chapter 2 would quickly reveal; and (d) medical narratives in additional media, especially film and television, could be addressed. On the other hand, I believe that this book has come to its appropriate resolution. What Henry James famously said about art applies, I believe, to rhetorical inquiry into the theory and interpretation of narrative: "relations stop nowhere" (5), and so one must find a way to bring one's work to a close. After 11 chapters, the time has come: I have unpacked the phrase "narrative as rhetoric" by identifying and explicating the principles of rhetorical theory, and I have also offered rhetorical treatments of nine key resources (character, progression, narration, dialogue, voice, perspective, time, space, and fictionality). I have also discussed how a rhetorical approach to those resources would need to adjust to account for graphic narrative as rhetoric. And of course, I have done a lot of close reading of a good range of narratives. Furthermore, I have a sense that deeper dives into the theoretical constructs and the individual narratives, while perhaps of interest to some readers, would have diminishing returns for more. Let be.

Another reason for stopping here is to hand things over to actual readers so that you can do your own reconfigurations of the book. What does the whole look like to you now that you've come to the end of it? What do you find most salient in its progression? Your answers to those questions are far more important than mine. Indeed, putting your interests first at this point constitutes reconfiguration as a productive dialogue between understanding and overstanding that can then be the basis for your springboarding. Have at it.

DOI: 10.4324/9781003018865-12

Finally, I want to thank you for engaging with this book to whatever degree you have. My sense of who you are and who you might be has influenced just about every aspect of my effort. At the same time, I realize that I may not have always successfully anticipated your interests and needs. Consequently, I invite you to send me your feedback at my Ohio State University email address: phelan.1@osu.edu. I want to hear from you because I believe that the best way to advance the project of Rhetorical Narrative Medicine is to treat all its proposals as works in progress. Onward!

Work Cited

James, Henry. *The Art of the Novel: Critical Prefaces*, edited by R.P. Black-mur. Chicago, IL: University of Chicago Press, 2011 [1934].

Glossary

This Glossary lists key terms in the book and defines them through the lens of rhetorical theory.[1]

ACTUAL AUDIENCE — Flesh-and-blood readers or viewers. Actual audience members who seek to join the AUTHORIAL AUDIENCE are RHETORICAL READERS. See also NARRATIVE AUDIENCE, NARRATEE.

AFFORDANCES — The features of a medium that lend themselves to particular ways of using it. For example, one of the features of comics is its dual track of verbal and visual communication. One of the affordances of the medium is the way it encourages interactions between those two tracks.

ANALEPSIS — In Gérard Genette's account, analepsis is any evocation of an event that took place prior to the point in time that the primary narrative has reached. This definition means that the more common term "flashback" is not an exact synonym for "analepsis" but rather identifies one frequently used kind. Flashback typically refers to the narration of an event or a series of events. Thus, in a statement such as "I love you more today than yesterday," most people would say that we have an analepsis ("more … than yesterday") but not a flashback.

AUDIENCE — See ACTUAL AUDIENCE, AUTHORIAL AUDIENCE, NARRATIVE AUDIENCE, NARRATEE, RHETORICAL READERS.

AUTHOR — The agent responsible for why the narrative text is the way it is and not some other way.

DOI: 10.4324/9781003018865-13

The agent who orchestrates the resources of narrative in order to accomplish some purposes in relation to a target audience. See also NARRATOR, DISTANCE.

AUTHORIAL AUDIENCE   The author's target audience. It is a hypothetical ideal, though usually based on the author's knowledge of some actual readers. In fiction, the authorial audience operates with the tacit knowledge that the characters and events are invented, synthetic constructs rather than real people and historical happenings. Nested within the authorial audience in fiction is the NARRATIVE AUDIENCE. See also RHETORICAL READERS.

AUTHORIAL DISCLOSURE ACROSS CONVERSATIONS   See DIALOGUE.

CHARACTER   The entity who acts or is acted upon in narrative. Character has three components: the MIMETIC (representation of a possible person); the THEMATIC (representative of a group or a set of ideas); and the SYNTHETIC (an artificial construct that performs a role in the larger construction of the narrative).

CHARACTER NARRATION   Telling in fiction or nonfiction by a participant in the events of the narrative. Rhetorical theory's alternative way of referring to what Genette calls homodiegetic narration.

CHRONOTOPE   Mikhail Bakhtin's term for the fusion of space and time in narrative; this fusion may be at the level of genre (novels of the road), or a governing concept (hospice), or a single passage.

COGNITIVE NARRATOLOGY   An approach to narrative that focuses on narrative as constructing mental models of storyworlds, including the cognitive activities of characters, and on the cognitive activities of audiences in reconstructing those mental models.

CONVERSATIONAL DISCLOSURE   See DIALOGUE.

CULTURAL NARRATIVE   A story that circulates widely within a given culture whose AUTHOR is not an individual agent but a larger collective entity, one that is at least a significant subgroup within that culture.

DEFICIENT NARRATION Reporting, interpreting, or evaluating by a narrator that is endorsed by the author but not by the actual audience. See also UNRELIABLE NARRATION.

DIALOGISM See HETEROGLOSSIA.

DIALOGUE Character-character conversations. This resource can function as an event and a means of narration. Authors use dialogue as a means of narration both in individual conversations and across two or more conversations. In the first use, called "conversational disclosure," characters and audiences typically share the same information. In the second, called "authorial disclosure across conversations," authors often invite audiences to make connections between or among the conversations that the characters cannot since they have not been present for all those conversations.

DISCOURSE The set of devices for telling a story, including VOICE (who speaks) and PERSPECTIVE (who perceives), and the handling of TEMPORALITY (see also ORDER, DURATION, and FREQUENCY). In structuralist conceptions of narrative, discourse is the "how" and STORY is the "what." See also STRUCTURALISM.

DISTANCE The relation between an author's implied views and the narrator's expressed views, especially along three axes of communication: about facts, characters, and events; about interpretations of those things; and about ethical evaluations of them. Distance exists along a spectrum from nonexistent or minimal to considerable to maximal. Distance is relevant to judgments of RELIABLE and UNRELIABLE NARRATION.

DOUBLE-VOICING An author's deployment of two VOICE(s) within a single utterance, with one implicitly commenting on the other. Irony works by double-voicing: there is the voice of the literal statement and the ironist's voice that undercuts it in some way. UNRELIABLE

	NARRATION, as a form of irony, also relies on double-voicing.
DURATION	Genette's term for the ratio between how long situations and events take to unfold in the raw materials of the story and how much text is devoted to their NARRATION. Variations in this ratio correspond to different narrative speeds; in order of increasing speed, these are PAUSE, SCENE, SUMMARY, and ELLIPSIS.
ELLIPSIS	Genette's term for the omission in the narration of events in the raw materials of the story. See also DURATION, GAPS.
ESSAY NARRATIVE	A hybrid form in which telling about change-over-time is juxtaposed with a teller's multiple reflections on something, their identification of problems and proposing solutions, or their making arguments.
EVENT	In the rhetorical definition of narrative "somebody telling somebody else ... that something happened," events are the somethings that happen. An event, then, is a happening, an occurrence, or a change of state.
EXPOSITION	Information about the context for the main events of a narrative, including backstory and current circumstances such as setting (time and place).
FEMINIST NARRATOLOGY	An approach to narrative that focuses on how issues of intersectional identity (e.g., gender, sexuality, class, race, disability) influence the construction, reception, and interpretation of narrative.
FICTIONALITY	From a rhetorical perspective, discourse in which somebody intentionally invents, projects, or otherwise directs somebody else to imagine non-actual states of affairs in order to influence that audience's understanding, beliefs, attitudes, or feelings about actual states of affairs and/or to persuade them to take some action about those states. See also NONFICTIONALITY.
FOCALIZATION	The answer to the question, "who perceives?" in the narrative discourse. Genette noted that the term "point of view" conflated two distinct aspects of narration: voice ("who

speaks?") and perception or focalization. Since Genette's separation of these two aspects, narrative theorists have been debating how best to distinguish among kinds of focalization. Rhetorical theory finds it most useful to work with the distinction between internal focalization (perception of a character) and external focalization (perception of a narrator), and to look at combinations of focalization and VOICE. See also PERSPECTIVE/POINT OF VIEW.

FREE INDIRECT DISCOURSE
Narration in which a character's discourse is embedded within or blends with a narrator's. The embedding is typically signaled by use of third-person rather than first-person narration and by the use of the past tense rather than the present. For example, Ernest Hemingway in "Hills Like White Elephants" reports the perceptions of one of the main characters this way: "They [the other people in the station] were all waiting reasonably for the train" (278).[2] The adverb "reasonably" is in the character's voice, but the "were" embeds it within the narrator's telling. If Hemingway were to use direct discourse, he'd shift to the present tense: "They are all waiting reasonably for the train."

FREQUENCY
Genette's term for the ratio between the number of times something is told and the number of times it occurs in the raw materials of the story. In *singulative* NARRATION, there is a one-to-one match between how many times an EVENT occurred and how many times it is told; in *iterative* narration, something that happens more than once is told once; and in *repetitive* narration, something that happens once is told multiple times (and, by extrapolation, in repetitive narration, something that happens N times is told N+X times).

GAPS
Omissions, incompleteness, or misalignments of various kinds. ELLIPSES are gaps in the narration of EVENTS. TENSIONS entail gaps between tellers and audiences. UNRELIABLE NARRATION involves gaps between authors and narrators.

GRAPHIC NARRATIVE | Somebody using the affordances of comics on some occasion and for some purposes to tell somebody else that something happened. See also NARRATIVE.

HETEROGLOSSIA | Bakhtin's term for the interplay of different sociolects within a society. He valued the novel as the genre that reflected—even required—such heteroglossia.

INSTABILITIES AND TENSIONS | Discordant situations that provide the basis for the textual dynamics of narrative progressions. Instabilities are part of plot dynamics, and they refer to discordant situations between or among characters; between a character and their situation; or within a character. Tensions are part of narratorial dynamics, and they refer to discordant situations between tellers and audiences. More specifically, tensions typically involve discrepancies in knowledge, beliefs, values, or judgments between narrators and narratees, narrators and authorial audience, or between authors and authorial audiences.

LYRIC NARRATIVE | A hybrid form in which plot is subordinated to the unfolding revelation of a particular situation, especially of a character in a situation and the feelings, ideas, and attitudes associated with that situation. In lyric narrative, situation is more important than character, whereas in PORTRAIT NARRATIVE character is more important than situation. In lyric narrative, the event sequences of plot either contribute relevant backstory or help reveal aspects of the character's situation.

MASTERPLOT | A general pattern of events shared by many individual narratives, such as the marriage plot. The master plots of a culture reveal a lot about that culture's common concerns and the way it prefers to address them.

METAREPRESENTATION | The idea that every statement (representation) comes from a source. Attending to metarepresentation entails tracking the sources of statements. When a statement becomes common knowledge (two plus two equals four), it can be detached from a source. In narrative, however, readers typically need to pay attention not just to what is said but also to who says it in order to judge its accuracy and authority (or so I say).

MINIMAL DEPARTURE, PRINCIPLE OF

Marie-Laure Ryan's idea that the storyworld of a fictional narrative conforms to the actual world of the reader, except about matters that the narrative explicitly marks as different. Thus, if the author does not say anything about such things as gravity or the speed of light, readers can assume that they operate the same way in the fictional world as they do in the actual world.

MIMETIC

A component of narrative construction and readerly interest involving a narrative's imitations of—or references to—the actual world, including such matters as characters functioning as possible people and events following the cause-effect logic of the extratextual world. The mimetic component is related to narrative's capacity for thick descriptions of character and events and for arousing strong emotions in actual audiences. See also CHARACTER, SYNTHETIC, THEMATIC.

MIMETIC-THEMATIC FEEDBACK LOOP

An interactive effect between the mimetic and thematic components of narrative best expressed in relation to authorial design and responses of AUTHORIAL AUDIENCES. Often authors will construct their narrative so that the more an authorial audience responds to the mimetic particulars of a character, a situation, or a set of events, the more the authorial audience recognizes their representative status and ideational import. And the more they recognize these generalizing aspects of the narrative, the more the authorial audience is likely to engage with the affective and the ethical dimensions of the mimetic representation.

NARRATEE

The audience addressed by the narrator. Sometimes the narratee is characterized, sometimes not. Sometimes the narratee functions as the narrator's ideal target audience, sometimes not. More generally, the narratee's relation to the NARRATOR, the NARRATIVE AUDIENCE, and the AUTHORIAL AUDIENCE can vary widely from one narrative to the next.

NARRATION   The processes and devices of telling. In print narrative, the narration operates along the single verbal track, while in comics narrative, narration operates along both the verbal and visual tracks and their interaction. See also DISCOURSE.

NARRATIVE   In informal usage, narrative is a synonym for STORY. In the rhetorical definition, narrative is somebody telling somebody else on some occasion and for some purpose(s) that something happened. "Something happened" is a key part of just about all definitions of narrative, referring to change over time.

NARRATIVE AUDIENCE   The observer role within the world of a fictional narrative, taken by the actual reader. In this sense, the narrative audience is the actual reader under an Invisibility Cloak, capable of observing without being observed. In this position, the narrative audience regards the characters and events as real and responds to them accordingly. The narrative audience position is nested within that of the AUTHORIAL AUDIENCE, giving actual readers who join the authorial audience a double consciousness (characters and events are real; characters and events are invented).

NARRATIVE DISCOURSE   See DISCOURSE, NARRATION.

NARRATIVE PROGRESSION   The movement of a narrative from beginning to end arising from a synthesis of TEXTUAL DYNAMIC and READERLY DYNAMICS. Textual dynamics refer to the introduction, complication, and resolution (often only partial) of a set of unstable relationships among CHARACTERS and/or between tellers and AUDIENCES, and readerly dynamics to the trajectory of the authorial audience's response to those textual dynamics. Rhetorical theory's interest in progression is more than an interest in the linear unfolding of narrative because it recognizes the authorial audience's dynamic, recursive activity in responding to the narrative's sequence of beginning, middle, and ending.

NARRATOLOGY | The study of the nature and workings of narrative. It is now a synonym for narrative theory, though the term originally designated a structuralist approach to narrative, devoted to writing a grammar of narrative patterned on the findings of structuralist linguistics. See also STRUCTURALISM.

NARRATOR | The explicit teller of a NARRATIVE. In rhetorical theory, the narrator is a resource that an author uses as part of their telling. Narrators perform three main functions: they report, they interpret, and they evaluate. See also NARRATORIAL DYNAMICS, UNRELIABLE NARRATION.

NARRATORIAL DYNAMICS | The trajectory of author—narrator—audience relationships across a PROGRESSION, marked by initiation (beginning), interaction (middle), and farewell (ending). The relationship may be stable or variable across the progression.

NONFICTIONALITY | From a rhetorical perspective, discourse in which somebody reports, interprets, evaluates, or otherwise engages with actual states of affairs in order to influence somebody else's understanding, beliefs, attitudes, or feelings about those states of affairs and/or to persuade them to take some action about those states. See also FICTIONALITY.

PARATEXT | Term coined by Genette to refer to materials accompanying a text, such as a title, authorial attribution, date of publication, preface, epigram, afterword, etc. These materials contextualize the narrative for its readers in multiple ways.

PAUSE | Genette's term for a type of DURATION in which the narration of events stops as the narration of other things, such as descriptions of space or philosophical reflections, continues.

PERSPECTIVE/POINT OF VIEW | Since Genette, narrative theory has discussed perspective and point of view under the heading of FOCALIZATION. Genette drew

a contrast between focalization and NAR-
RATION to distinguish between who sees
or perceives and who speaks in a narrative,
respectively. See also VOICE.

PLOT DYNAMICS   The sequence of events in a narrative and its
underlying logic. Plot proceeds from begin-
ning to middle to ending through a pattern of
instability—complication—resolution (though
resolution is often only partial). Plot dynamics
generate READERLY DYNAMICS and can
be influenced by them. See also PROGRES-
SION, NARRATORIAL DYNAMICS,
TEXTUAL DYNAMICS.

PORTRAIT NARRATIVE   A hybrid form in which narrative is present
but subordinated to the revelation of char-
acter. Where narrative is concerned with
change over time, portrait narrative is concerned with gradually disclosing the key
traits of a possible or actual person.

PRINCIPLE OF MINIMAL   See MINIMAL DEPARTURE, PRINCI-
DEPARTURE   PLE OF.

PROGRESSION   The overall movement of a narrative from
beginning through middle to ending. It is a
synthesis of TEXTUAL DYNAMICS and
READERLY DYNAMICS as well as the
underlying logic governing that synthesis.
Understanding progression can be a valuable
way of identifying a narrative's purpose(s).

PROLEPSIS   In Genette's model, the evocation before
the fact of an event that will take place later
in the primary narrative. Flashforward is one
type of prolepsis.

READERLY DYNAMICS   The trajectory of RHETORICAL READ-
ERS' responses to the TEXTUAL DYNAM-
ICS, typically involving cognitive, affective,
ethical, and aesthetic layers. An author's sense
of readerly dynamics can influence their construction of the textual dynamics.

RELIABLE NARRATION   Reporting, interpreting, or evaluating by a
narrator that is endorsed by the author. See
also DEFICIENT NARRATION, UNRE-
LIABLE NARRATION.

RHETORICAL READERS   Actual readers who seek to become members
of the author's target audience. See also

SCENE | AUTHORIAL AUDIENCE, NARRA-TIVE AUDIENCE, NARRATEE.

In Genette's model, scenic presentation is a narrative speed or mode of DURATION in which one can assume a direct equivalence between how long it takes for things to happen in the world of the story and how long it takes the NARRATOR—or how much textual space is required—to recount those happenings.

SPACE | The environment(s) in which the events of a narrative happen. Following Marie-Laure Ryan, we can identify several aspects of space in narrative: (a) spatial frames—the places in which events occur such as rooms, buildings, streets, parks, and so on; (b) story space—the sum total of the narrative's spatial frames; (c) setting—the spatial-temporal context for the narrative; (d) storyworld—the larger world containing the story space, completed by the reader's imagination as informed by relevant cultural knowledge; and (e) narrative universe—the actual world constructed by the text plus all the other worlds projected or imagined by narrators or characters.

STORY | In common usage, a synonym for NAR-RATIVE. In structuralist narratology, the what of narrative, its events and existents—character, events, and place. The events in chronological order constitute the story abstracted from the discourse. See also STRUCTURALISM.

STRUCTURALISM | An approach to literary and cultural analysis, especially prominent in the 1960s and 1970s, that used structuralist linguistics as a model for studying a wide range of cultural expressions as rule-governed ways of combining basic building blocks (e.g., phonemes, words, sentences) into larger structures. Structuralist narratology took on the task of writing a grammar of narrative, that is, of identifying the fundamental elements of stories and the ways they could be combined. The project's founding move is to divide narrative into a what (story) and a how (discourse). It then identifies the elements of story (primarily events, characters, and space) and the elements of discourse (narration and temporality), analyzes them further, and then considers how these elements come together in the structure of a narrative.

SYNTHETIC   A component of narrative construction and readerly interest concerned with a narrative, and its parts, including characters and events, as constructed objects—something artificial rather than natural, something fashioned rather than found.

SUMMARY   Genette's term for a narrative speed or mode of DURATION faster than SCENE but slower than ELLIPSIS; summaries can vary in how detailed they are, but they are always more condensed than representations of SCENES.

TENSIONS   See INSTABILITIES AND TENSIONS.

THEMATIC   A component of narrative and readerly interest involving the ideational, ethical, and ideological dimensions of the narrative, including its handling of character as representing a larger group or set of ideas.

TEMPORALITY   The handling of time in narrative, especially in the narrative discourse. Genette builds his categories of ORDER, DURATION, and FREQUENCY by attending to the relations between time in the raw materials of the narrative (what he calls STORY) and time in discourse itself.

TEXTUAL DYNAMICS   The internal logic of a text's progression consisting of PLOT DYNAMICS in combination with NARRATORIAL DYNAMICS.

TIME   See TEMPORALITY.

UNRELIABLE   A mode of NARRATION in which the
NARRATION   author does not endorse the narrator's reporting, interpreting, or evaluating of characters and events. Unreliable narration may have estranging or bonding effects. Estranging effects increase the DISTANCE (ethical, epistemological, affective, or otherwise) between the narrator and the authorial audience, while bonding effects close that distance.

| VISION | See FOCALIZATION; PERSPECTIVE; POINT OF VIEW. |
| VOICE | The answer to the question, who is speaking? Rhetorical theory adds that voice is the synthesis of style, rhythm, tone, and values. See also FOCALIZATION, NARRATION. |

Notes

1 Some of the entries here draw on the glossary that David Herman, Brian McHale, and I co-authored for *Teaching Narrative Theory* (MLA Publications, 2010).
2 Hemingway, Ernest. "Hills Like White Elephants." In *The Short Stories of Ernest Hemingway*, 273–278. New York: Scribner, 1953.

Index